Advance praise for WYLDE ON HEALTH

"Bryce makes all of us wildly passionate about our health and shares accessible insights and achievable action steps to bring youthful vigour into all our lives." **Mehmet Oz**, MD, Professor and vice chair, surgery, NY Presbyterian/Columbia

"Bryce Wylde gives sensible, medically sound advice in this comprehensive manual on health, covering everything from optimum dietary habits to appropriate use of diagnostic tests and natural remedies for common problems. If you want to take greater control of your health, this book will be a great help." **Andrew Weil**, MD, author of *8 Weeks to Optimum Health*

"I am a doctor, and a nut about fitness. I want to live as long and as functional a life as possible, and constantly educate myself to make that happen. We don't know everything about the human body, but we know more than ever before. My friend Bryce Wylde has written a book that should be in your home today and will make you smarter about your own body. If you are wild about your health and want to take control, turn the page." **Sanjay Gupta**, MD, CNN Chief Medical Correspondent

"For anyone who doubted the science behind alternative therapies and their effectiveness, this book will help them understand the many options natural medicine can provide to improve and maintain their overall health." **Randy Boyer**, co-founder, The Healthy Shopper Inc., co-author of *Unjunk Your Junk Food*

"Bryce Wylde is one of our most trusted health experts, and the state-of-the-art self-testing covered in *Wylde on Health* is the missing key to unlocking the mystery of chronic health challenges we face today. This book is a must-read for anyone ready to take the[illegible] vitality to the next level." **Julie Daniluk**, RHN, au[illegible] *That Heal Inflammation*

"Bryce Wylde's professional experience as [illegible] clinician, coupled with his passion for researc[illegible] make *Wylde on Health* a must-read for any[illegible] a healthy lifestyle." **Andrea Donsky**, RHN, crea[illegible] NaturallySavvy.com, co-author of *Unjunk Your Junk Food*

"*Wylde on Health* paves the way to the emerging future, to aid you in having the healthiest, happiest and most energized life possible." **Sam Graci**, author of *The Five Keys to Amazing Energy*

"In an age dominated by pharmaceuticals and marketing hype, *Wylde on Health* uncovers—in layman's lingo—the all-too-often complex and confusing subject of how to get healthy fast by using the most natural and proven means accessible to us. Bryce has done all the legwork—now all you have to do is read the book!" **Brad King**, MS, MFS, nutritional researcher and author of *Beer Belly Blues*

"Bryce Wylde's book is a comprehensive, intelligently written and invaluable guide to natural and preventive medicine which, as he rightly states, should never be considered 'alternative.' This science-based and practical information will reassure and empower individuals to control many aspects of their own health, which is the only path to a healthy life. I will be recommending this book." **Jozef Krop**, MD, HD, author of *Healing the Planet: One Patient at a Time*

"In the often confusing and hype-filled world of natural health, Bryce Wylde stands apart as a trusted authority. He has once again synthesized thousands of scientific papers from various medical disciplines into a concise, reader-friendly resource. With the unique insight that only he can provide, Bryce brilliantly weaves together his clinical, research and broadcasting experiences, engaging the reader from cover to cover." **Alan C. Logan**, ND, co-author of *Your Brain on Nature*

"Bryce Wylde brilliantly separates fact from junk science, explaining how to use specific health-promoting foods, supplements and simple home tests to reclaim your health, live longer and complement medical treatment for many common health problems and diseases of our time. A must-read for every health-conscious person." **James Meschino**, DC, MS, ND, author of *The Meschino Optimal Living Program*

"*Wylde on Health* is a must-read: the perfect guide for those looking to achieve optimal health naturally." **Joey Shulman**, DC, registered nutritionist, author of *The Metabolism-Boosting Diet*

"As a pre-eminent integrative medicine expert, Bryce Wylde has an encyclopedic knowledge that spans topics as diverse as digestion, anti-aging medicine, cardiovascular and neurodegenerative diseases. *Wylde on Health* is an invaluable resource to help you live and perform at your best!" **Robb Wolf**, author of *The Paleo Solution*

WYLDE ON HEALTH

YOUR BEST CHOICES IN THE WORLD OF NATURAL HEALTH

BRYCE WYLDE

Bsc, RNC, DHMHS, HOMEOPATH

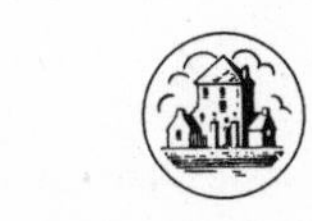

RANDOM HOUSE CANADA

PUBLISHED BY RANDOM HOUSE CANADA

 Published in 2012 by Random House Canada, a division of Random House of Canada Limited, Toronto. Distributed in Canada by Random House of Canada Limited.

www.randomhouse.ca

This book is intended as a reference volume only and not as a medical manual. It is not intended as a substitute for any treatment that may have been prescribed by a doctor. The author is not responsible for your specific health or allergy needs that may require medical supervision, or for any adverse reactions to the recipes contained in this book.

The recommendations in this book are generic, since nutritional needs vary depending on age, sex, and health status. If you suspect that you have a serious medical problem, the author strongly recommends seeking proper medical treatment.

Library and Archives Canada Cataloguing in Publication

Wylde, Bryce
Wylde on health : your best choices in the world of natural health / Bryce Wylde.

Includes index.
Also issued in electronic format.
ISBN 978-0-307-35587-4

1. Nutrition. 2. Health. 3. Alternative medicine. I. Title.

RA784.W95 2012 613.2 C2012-902108-3

Text and cover design by Leah Springate
Cover image: Curtis Lantinga, Photographer
Printed and bound in the United States of America

10 9 8 7 6 5 4 3 2 1

I dedicate this to you, who are interested in discovering the power of the body's innate ability to heal itself. I dedicate this to you, who—once healed—are interested in *remaining* healthy. But I wouldn't have written this at all if it weren't for the influence of my own mother who introduced me at an early age to the incredible healing powers of Mother Nature.

CONTENTS

FOREWORD

Bryce Wylde is no ordinary homeopath. He is a practitioner with an exceptional palette of skills: not only is he a visionary proponent of integrative health, a charismatic media personality, a successful author and an astute entrepreneur, he is also a sound clinician and interpreter of the latest science of natural medicines. Moreover, he is a dedicated family man, a sportsman and an authentically nice guy who really does practise what he preaches.

I first met Bryce when he and his film crew arrived with a flourish at a downtown Toronto executive health clinic in 2008. He was there to submit to a full four-hour head-to-toe medical exam that included some unique genetic testing coupled with lifestyle counselling, an experience that many others would go through when it became a feature on his TV show *Wylde on Health*. Fortuitously, I was to be his doctor.

I had caught episodes of his television series and thought that he and I might engage in some interesting discussions, but I was unprepared for the synergies we discovered we had—and for the friendship that has since developed. Subsequent to that first meeting I have made guest appearances on his live TV series, where I've been amazed at Bryce's ability to handle verbose guests with aplomb, ask the right questions at the right time, navigate multiple, complex technologies (teleprompters, producers speaking into his headset while he interacts with telephone callers and BlackBerry texters), and through it all to remain calm and in control.

While Bryce and I originated from opposite ends of the health-care spectrum—I started from the allopathic or conventional medicine side as an internal medicine specialist, and he from the CAM (complementary alternative medicine) side—we are now both solidly planted in the middle. We share the conviction that the future of health care must and will be a thoughtful integration of evidence-based Western medicine with CAM practices, which are also increasingly evidence-based, and are very often founded on thousands of years of human use. We also concur that health is best achieved when patients' care is personalized and they are active participants in it.

Western medicine has excelled in the areas of high-technology diagnostics and treatment, and it applies its skills to particularly good effect in the management of acute illnesses. However, it is reductionist by nature, and focuses mechanistically on the workings of our bodies at a molecular level. Considerations of spirit, consciousness, humanity and the interconnections of sentient beings are not often part of typical patient–physician discussions. For many people, it is these aspects of patient care that attract them to CAM. The practitioners of complementary medicine—doctors of naturopathy, chiropractic, traditional Chinese medicine, Ayurveda and homeopathy, to name a few—are adept at establishing alliances with patients by adopting a "whole health" stance and by assisting them to manage chronic illnesses. With conditions such as diabetes, depression or chronic pain, a therapeutic approach that incorporates lifestyle and preventive perspectives can be an important complement to prescription medications. It is clear that the integrative approach is resonating with North Americans, with recent studies showing that more than 40 percent of our population visits one or more CAM practitioners concurrently with their conventional medical doctors.

The vision of full collaboration amongst the entire spectrum of health providers led Bryce to found one of the first truly integrated clinics in Canada, which has enjoyed considerable success. I wholeheartedly endorse his tenets that good health, well-being and longevity depend on four components: 1) fitness of the body 2) nutrition (including supplements where indicated) 3) fitness of the mind (including stress management, regular contemplative practice such as yoga, tai chi or meditation) and 4) connectivity, defined as self-awareness and positive relationships with one's family, community and the environment. When these four legs of the "table of health" are balanced through a personalized and participatory approach, the table stands solid. But paying attention to only one or two legs leads the table to wobble and collapse.

In this book Bryce consolidates his vast knowledge and clinical experience with patients, addresses their concerns and offers his expert advice on how best to establish a "whole health" way of life. This includes specific recommendations on the diagnostic tools available to assess one's current health status, as well as detailed information about the natural health products (NHPs) and functional medicines that can restore and maintain good health. Research from the nutraceutical and functional medicine industries is vast, and the volume of studies is increasing rapidly. Few health practitioners have as complete a grasp of this research as Bryce Wylde does. From algae to xenobiotics and everything in between, *Wylde on Health* walks us through what is potentially helpful and what is not, in a concise and unbiased way. While it is written for laypersons and is easy to read, Bryce has put considerable effort into backing up the credibility of the science and strength of evidence behind his advice. He has even developed his own rating system that uses five criteria—assessment of claims, potential benefits, strength of evidence, the cost, and the safety of the most important NHPs—to generate a percentage score. Like picking a fine wine at the liquor store, it is intuitive and easy to use this rating scale to compare supplements that are currently available in pharmacies and health food stores, and to choose the one(s) that are right for you. This book will appeal equally to those who are suffering from chronic ailments and those who are well but wish to be proactive about health promotion and disease prevention. For budding scientists, there are chemical equations (but only a few) and explanations of the most recent and relevant genomics testing that enables a personalized medicine approach.

Along the way *Wylde on Health* provides concise action plans for healthier living in all of our major organ systems and all four legs of our health table. From information on dietary and bowel habits to recommendations on how to improve our sexual lives or use biofeedback to de-stress, there is truly something here for everyone. Enjoy!

Dr. Tim Cook, MD, FRCPC, MPH, CD

CHAPTER 1

—

INTRODUCTION

It was a fine, warm afternoon in May 2008, when I stopped at Starbucks for a self-indulgent second coffee before heading up to the old Citytv broadcast facilities. It was a smell-the-flowers kind of day, except, of course, there were few flowers in the vicinity of 299 Queen Street. I ran into Leila, my assistant producer, who'd come out for a coffee of her own.

"This should be a good one," she said.

"Agreed. See you up there."

The transition from full-time clinician to part-time broadcaster had been a pretty smooth one for me. I'd used the first six months to march through the core topics of integrative medicine—supplements, vitamins, minerals, diet, exercise—and had begun to consider where I was going to take the program from there. I was relatively green as a broadcaster, and none of the big names—Mehmet Oz, Andrew Weil, Sanjay Gupta, Deepak Chopra—had yet appeared on the show. We'd had a stream of guest experts, but none of them were such celebrities in their fields. One of the highlights of the show at that time had always been the interaction with viewers, whom I invited to call in during every show. I enjoyed talking to and listening to people about their health concerns and I was able to use the exchanges to first understand what was on people's minds and then to gradually define for my audience what my understanding of good medicine was—and what it wasn't.

I walked down the long corridor and past the sports desk, where we had the little *Wylde on Health* set in a corner of the newsroom. My producer, Darren Weir, was on the phone when I arrived.

"Yes, any time," he was saying. "As long as he's here thirty minutes before we go on air . . . certainly . . . no, I know that. I know how tight his schedule is. Don't worry, we'll have him in and out of here in no time."

He hung up, smiled.

"Guy's got an army of handlers," he said.

Apparently landing Dr. Sha Zhi Gang was more of a coup than I'd realized. I'd received a promotional package from his PR people some months before and filed it away until we'd covered a bit more ground. Now the time was right. Traditional Chinese medicine (TCM to the cognoscenti) is one of the founts from which integrative medicine flows and this Dr. Sha was not only a practitioner of TCM but a physician trained and licensed in China. It couldn't get much more integrative than that. The week before, I'd watched a documentary and discovered that before he moved to Toronto in 1990, he'd been the lead acupuncturist for the World Health Organization and for leaders in the Philippines, Taiwan and China. He was a master in tai chi, qigong, I Ching, kung fu and feng shui. He had a master's degree in hospital administration from the University of the Philippines. He'd been named Qigong Master of the Year at the Fifth World Congress on qigong in San Francisco, and in 2006 New Jersey had presented him with the Martin Luther King Jr. Commemorative Commission Award.

I flipped through my notes. "We've got our first real celebrity," I said.

"Yeah." Darren was fiddling with a light. "And he comes with great b-roll."

The b-roll is auxiliary visual material that the producers can run during the course of a show. Dr. Sha's b-roll was boggling. There was stuff on how natural techniques were curing people in China. There were scenes of crowds—*crowds*—of Westerners listening raptly to his lectures, crowds of Westerners singing some sort of Chinese songs, crowds of Westerners holding their hands in identical positions. I didn't know what any of this meant, but I've got a lot of respect for the discipline and utility of the martial arts. And a grandmaster of feng shui who was also a hospital administrator and a physician? It was fine with me.

I didn't see anything about soul transplants. I didn't see anything about organ downloads. The words "personality cult" were never mentioned.

Dr. Sha Zhi Gang was a robust, genial—even jovial—gentleman in early middle age. He shook my hand with vigour and seemed utterly relaxed in the sometimes intimidating environment of a TV studio. He laughed heartily at my feeblest bons mots as we set up the mikes and got ourselves in place. In fact, he laughed quite a lot of the time.

I was a bit worried about Dr. Sha's heavy Mandarin accent—several times I didn't quite understand what he was saying—but apparently a lot of other people did and my job was really just to ask questions. I knew a little about the man's varied career in medicine, but it was traditional Chinese medicine that I wanted to talk about.

We were on. I read the introduction and we exchanged the on-air pleasantries before moving on to acupuncture and the like. In the second segment I was delighted to find Sha ready and willing to demonstrate TCM procedures. He took my pulse and said nice things about it but his centrepiece was the reading of my tongue. A Western physician can tell a couple of things from a patient's tongue, but for a TCM practitioner, it's supposed to be an open book. I won't say I was flattered, but I admit I was pleased—maybe relieved—when Dr. Sha had finished his examination and laughed out loud.

"You got great tongue," he said.

Out of the corner of my eye, I could see Darren and Leila smirking. I have something of a reputation as a talker.

"You got very clean organs," he said.

Now, I try to keep my organs as clean as the next person, maybe cleaner, but it was awe-inspiring to think that a man was so experienced, he could literally see into me through my tongue.

"Wow," I said.

The final segment of the show was the one where I invite people to call in with questions for me and/or my guest. Now I took the first call.

"Hello, Dr. Wylde," a soft-voiced lady said. "Hello, Dr. Sha. My name's Evelyn and I'm calling because I have pancreatic cancer."

There was nothing irregular in my screeners allowing a call through from a person suffering from a dreadful disease that is almost universally fatal. I'd instructed them to do so, because these people are understandably desperate and it was a chance for me to make the point that "alternative" medicine—as I and others I respect practise it—doesn't deal in miracles. We're not in the business of curing the incurable. But it's also a chance to illustrate how natural products and techniques can improve the quality of life remaining to such people—and sometimes help to extend that life.

I was starting to explain just that when Dr. Sha smiled broadly and held up his hand.

"Please, Dr. Wylde," he said. "I would like please to perform a soul surgery."

You know, I may not quite have heard him correctly. The Chinese accent can be a challenge for the unfamiliar ear.

"Sure," I said, with some hesitation.

Dr. Sha stood and began a low chant in his native language. He began to wave his hands in wide arcs and his voice rose to a crescendo. I looked desperately at Darren and was furious to see him laughing. Why hadn't they ever installed that big red button I'd asked for? (The one that would drop a guest through trap doors from under them in the case of a horrible fail!) Finally, in a closing frenzy, Dr. Sha flung his hands in the direction of the camera and issued a final command—in English.

"Transmission!" he shouted.

I believe we were to understand that a new pancreas was on its way or had perhaps already been delivered. Dr. Sha sat down.

"You better," he said to the camera, seemingly exhausted.

"Thank you," Evelyn said.

There was a moment of silence.

"Um, Dr. Sha," I said. "I'd like to talk a bit about Chinese herbs."

Afterwards, Dr. Sha expressed his gratitude for this chance to demonstrate his skills and broaden his public. He put his hand on my chest and held it there a moment.

"You very old soul," he said. "Ten thousand one hundred years."

"Gosh," I said.

"Even me, I only twelve thousand three hundred," he said.

For weeks after this broadcast we received calls from viewers hoping Dr. Sha was still somewhere around. It seemed he held an unshakeable appeal for some of my audience, who saw more in his miracles than in my own rather humble claims, and the advice I offered based on integrative medicine. And in fact it was months before I felt I'd clearly re-established for my viewers the boundaries within alternative medicine, the boundaries between alternative and conventional medicine, and the boundaries between good and bad medicine. That's something I want to discuss in this chapter.

NAVIGATING YOUR HEALTH CHOICES

I believe the path I'm treading is a worthy one. I believe in listening to others—not just researchers and broadcasters and doctors, but ordinary folks with ordinary health problems. During my tenure as the host of *Wylde on Health*, I answered over a thousand calls and e-mails live on the air. I'm planning a new show now and I continue to interact. I exchange information with visitors to my website, I sit up at night reading scientific papers, I scan health blogs and monitor posts from patients and practitioners both. And yes, I follow Twitter trends, which is one of the ways I keep tabs on the buzz in my field (and you can follow me: @wyldeonhealth). Meanwhile, I administer and attend a busy full-time health clinic, where I'm a health practitioner with my own roster of patients.

One way or another, that's a lot of listening, so it won't come as a surprise that I've formed a pretty clear impression of what people care about when it comes to complementary and alternative health solutions—how could I not?—and that overall impression is, in a nutshell, what's behind this book. As far as I can manage it between two covers, I've tried to bring together my best evidence-based answers to the questions that are on the top of people's minds—people like you, the informed and health-conscious.

Before we begin, I want to say a little about my practice and where it fits in the swarm of terminology that describes non-conventional medicine. The clinic where I serve as director, just north of Toronto, is home to a team of physicians, homeopaths, naturopaths, nutritionists, chiropractors, physiotherapists, massage therapists, an audiologist and dentists who work together across disciplines to take care of our patients' health. At the clinic, we provide services in complementary alternative medicine within a medical setting that emphasizes *integrative care* and eschews an "instead of," "either-or" way of thinking in favour of an approach that engages with our patients and allows them to become part of the decision-making process. We employ evidence-based natural medicine and run human clinical trials to advance research in complementary alternative therapies. We provide natural solutions—lifestyle, diet, antioxidant therapies, botanical medicine, I.V. therapies, homeopathics, nutraceuticals and functional medicine testing—that conventional medicine simply cannot offer within its standard parameters. Nonetheless, as a philosophy, integrative medicine does not constitute a blanket endorsement of every form of alternative medicine. And because there isn't yet a perfect consensus on some of the terminology in this area, let me take a minute to set out our understanding of these various but not unrelated terms.

Conventional Medicine

There is a common perception that "alternative" clinicians, working outside the standard medical field, fail to grasp the achievements of science. There are no doubt such people, but I and my colleagues are assiduous in our appreciation for conventional medicine's strengths. I personally hold conventional medicine and its good doctors, specialists, nurses and pharmacists in the highest regard. Let me go further. Judged by the standards of scientific research, much of the alternative approach is not yet proven. There's a caveat though: where most conventional medicine *is* scientifically validated, some is *not.* I encourage patients to approach all medical situations with their eyes and ears open, and I encourage conventional medical doctors to keep their minds open too.

Alternative Medicine

To my way of thinking, any therapy that is typically excluded by conventional medicine, and that patients use *instead of* conventional medicine, can be termed "alternative medicine." It's a blanket term that includes many old and new therapies such as acupuncture, herbology, homeopathy and iridology. Generally speaking, alternative therapies are derived more directly from nature, and are usually less expensive and less invasive than conventional therapies.

Complementary Alternative Medicine (CAM)

When alternative medicine is employed in conjunction with conventional medicine, we say that the physician is practising "complementary" medicine. My practice model is an example. A practical instance of CAM might be using arnica to reduce swelling and bruising in the case of a casted broken bone, or glutamine to prevent muscle and weight loss when undergoing chemotherapy in cancer. In fact, L-glutamine has been shown to increase the chemotherapeutic effect of cancer medication by more than 25 percent. Another example might be the use of essential fatty acids from fish oil and coenzyme Q10 (CoQ10) concomitant to the use of cholesterol-lowering medication—fish oil to improve HDL (good cholesterol) levels and CoQ10 to offset the side effects of the cholesterol medication.

Integrative Medicine

The National Center for Complementary Alternative Medicine (NC-CAM), part of the U.S. National Institutes of Health (NIH), defines integrative medicine as "combining mainstream medical therapies and CAM therapies for which there is some high-quality scientific evidence of safety and effectiveness."

True integrative medicine incorporates only scientifically validated therapies from both conventional and CAM systems. It considers only the best of the best and most rigorously tested evidence-based approaches, while endorsing the partnership between patient and practitioner as essential in the healing process. Integrative medicine is the appropriate use of conventional and alternative methods to facilitate the body's innate healing response. Integrative medicine considers all factors that influence health, wellness and disease—mind, body, spirit and community—and embraces a philosophy that neither rejects conventional medicine nor accepts alternative therapies uncritically. It is the official position of the NC-CAM at the NIH that good medicine should be inquiry driven, open to new paradigms and based in good science. Integrative medicine can also be characterized by the use of natural, effective, less invasive interventions whenever possible.

My own model for clinical testing is essentially preventive and considers a patient's functional parameters, micronutrient status, toxin load, genomics and subclinical deficiencies. My philosophy is that I don't search for a needle in a haystack—that is, I don't rely on one seemingly pivotal factor to justify treatment—but I do rule in or out as many factors as possible through clinical history and biological sampling or screening. I hope you'll find such a philosophy reflected in this book, as I offer to you some of the same methodologies I apply in my own practice. Our first step will be to discover how healthy you actually are, then we'll look at what you can do to become healthier in a variety of ways, and finally how you can hold on to those gains.

I don't simply rely on objective parameters. In practice I also rely on my patients' individual, subjective experiences. Again, *listening* to my patients, hearing the details of their stories with empathy and my fullest attention and keeping a detailed record of their subjective symptoms is the first key to my approach.

And because I hold scientifically validated clinical knowledge in the highest regard, assessment by testing is the second key. I've seen a great many patients over the years and have selected a roster of laboratories that offer a range of testing for human biological samples. I am aligned with the following local and international laboratories: Gamma Dynacare, Genova Diagnostics, Neuro Science, Pharmasan, Metametrix, Rocky Mountain Labs, Axys Analytics, Doctors Data, Navigenics, Genovations, Clifford Consulting, Counsyl, Entero Lab and Quicksilver Scientific, to name a few.

MY PRACTICE. MY PATIENTS.

I learn by reading, just as we all do. But the most valuable advice I have to pass on to you is drawn from my experience with my patients. To my formal training I've added years of personal clinical experience with natural remedies, tests, lifestyle and nutrition. That's where theory is proven or rejected. So before we get down to the core of my message, allow me to follow a patient and illustrate how my practice actually works.

Nick R. is a thirty-two-year-old married man living in suburban Toronto. He runs a modest but successful business as a general contractor and has designed and built some handsome houses. For the last five years, Nick, who is a light smoker, has been increasingly troubled by shortness of breath, tightness in his chest and wheezing—worsening in the spring and after meals. He finally finds the time to see his doctor and his doctor orders a pulmonary function test that confirms a diagnosis of asthma. Nick is forty pounds overweight and already takes a statin medication because of high serum cholesterol levels. His doctor prescribes a rescue inhaler (Salbutamol/Ventolin), an Advair discus and a comprehensive allergy skin scratch test—he's a doctor whose approach is thorough. The inhaler provides some relief from the asthma symptoms but Nick is still experiencing shortness of breath and tightness in his chest and feels increasingly anxious and moody. His doctor is a bit stumped but refers Nick to a respiratory specialist. The appointment is in October. This is May.

Nick's sister-in-law is a patient of mine and she talks him into contacting my office. During our first interview, I explain to Nick that we're not going to be undoing any of the treatments prescribed by his doctor. Our first goal will be to understand something about "the whole Nick." Then, and only then, we can perhaps work together to develop a customized action plan that involves effective natural approaches.

I run some tests that identify immune status, indicate some food sensitivities, and uncover vitamin D and CoQ10 deficiencies. Through a genomic assessment, I determine Nick's predisposition to chronic inflammation (specifically, a set of mutations on genes that control inflammation—even more specifically, the TNF-alpha and TH-2 cytokines). Through further testing, I'm able to determine that Nick has a high urinary output of the neurotransmitter dopamine, suggesting extreme stress and anxiety. My plan of action is to get him on the right vitamins, herbs, homeopathics and antioxidants (at the right doses) to balance his immune system, lower his reactivity to environmental triggers, balance his dopamine and decrease his stress—the last factor inevitably contributing to the immune-suppressing levels of the hormone cortisol. I then go on to specify the right diet to match his immune function to his allergies and sensitivities. Here's what Nick and I agree on and why:

I recommend incorporating a chlorella supplement because it may reduce inflammation specific to his genetic expression. I recommend 5,000 IU vitamin D daily due to his deficiency in this important vitamin and its ability to support the immune system. I recommend 100mg of CoQ10 twice daily to offset the side effects of his cholesterol medication. I recommend theanine to help relax him and help balance dopamine levels, which will also reduce his cravings for cigarettes. (He's only going to stop when he's ready.)

Nutritionally, I recommend incorporating maitake mushrooms (because they can stimulate the production and activity of natural killer [NK] cells that may help protect Nick against lung cancer). I suggest hijiki algae, which can facilitate the release of the TNF-α—again offsetting one of his genetic glitches. Also on his new menu are spirulina, propolis and probiotic-rich yogurt, all of which work to balance his immune system.

Predisposition to chronic inflammation is one of Nick's underlying genetic weaknesses and his lifestyle contributes to it so I recommend that he include coconut oil, fish oils, flax seed oil and nuts and seeds to inhibit the production and release of interleukin-6 (known to contribute to asthma).

Choline, found plentifully in egg yolk, is an essential nutrient related to the water-soluble B-complex vitamins. Nick could use more of that since choline appears to decrease the severity of asthma symptoms, the number of symptomatic days and the need to use bronchodilators. His doctor's referral to an allergist didn't reveal any specific allergies on the skin scratch test—including eggs—but because he could still have sensitivities to foods that we hadn't yet tested for, I avoid recommending eggs in his diet and put him on supplemental choline, which would provide him with a therapeutic dose that he'd not get from eggs alone.

I also prescribe a resin extract from the *Boswellia serrata* tree that has been found to have anti-inflammatory effects. Evidence suggests that boswellia is effective as a chronic therapy for asthma that, unlike the popular non-steroidal anti-inflammatory drugs (NSAIDs), does not cause gastrointestinal irritation with long-term use.

Finally, since certain breathing patterns in asthma patients can have adverse effects on the airways and lead to symptom exacerbation, and because affective and anxiety disorders are more common among people with asthma, I recommend a biofeedback program for Nick. Research has demonstrated that heart-rate-variability biofeedback has strong long-term influences on pulmonary function.

By the fall of that year, Nick was a new person. He had lost over thirty pounds and was off his prescription medication, needing only to rely on the Ventolin rescue inhaler on the very odd occasion. His new focus on healthy foods and the fact that he'd stopped smoking had resulted in his doctor taking him off of his cholesterol medication. He was able to stop CoQ10 supplementation too. His vitamin D levels read perfectly normal three months later and he was able to maintain at a dose of 2,000 IU/day. He no longer gets frequent colds or flu, his chest is lighter, he has no shortness of breath, and in fact takes the stairs instead of the elevator anytime he can. He reports that his skin has cleared up, his energy improved, concentration is much better, and his anxiety has disappeared, thanks largely to the biofeedback techniques.

Nick, of course, knew something was wrong and he sought help. Every sensible person should do so—although many men have to experience a heart attack or lose a limb before they'll admit to a problem. But even if you feel you're "one hundred and ten percent," you may still find the next chapter worth reading. Before we consider getting healthier and then staying healthy, let's ask ourselves, really, how healthy are we now?

CHAPTER 2

HOW HEALTHY ARE WE?

I spend a great deal of time in front of TV cameras, where I'm often in conversation with members of the public. Many of the people I speak to and hear from are there because there's something about natural and alternative medicine that stirs their interest. Based on what they read and perhaps on how they're feeling, they suspect that they are not as healthy as they could be, and that the root of the problem may be our modern lifestyle and diet.

Take the idea of "enriched" food, for example. Manufacturers want health-conscious consumers to believe that any food that is labelled as enriched is a healthier choice. In the case of wheat, if you strip the grain of many of its nutrients, take away its fibre, bleach the heck out of it and then pulverize it into a fine dust to maximize the speed at which the carbohydrate content enters the bloodstream as sugar, you get white flour—North America's staple food. Throw a few bits of nutrition back in for good measure—a little vitamin A, some vitamin B, some folic acid, perhaps some tiny amount of reconstituted fibre—whatever makes for good package marketing at the time—and you've got enriched flour. Add some water, salt and baking powder, and you've got bread. A lot of people are starting to suspect that eating processed foods—including most enriched foods—on a regular basis can result in malnutrition in the midst of plenty. And they're right. It's not even that unusual for a North American nowadays to be living with an absolute clinical nutrient deficiency. For example, it is estimated that 75 percent of North Americans are deficient in vitamin D and millions of others are very low in this nutrient that scientists have agreed is crucial to bone, immune system and nervous system health.

The above example is just one among many I could highlight. Over the years of interactions with patients and viewers I've noticed that health concerns tend to cluster around certain subjects. For each of these, people want to understand more about the underlying mechanisms, more about the problems that can arise when those mechanisms go wrong, more about how they can assess their own status and, of course, what they can do about it.

I'm going to devote this chapter to understanding and assessment—that is, testing. In the next chapter I'll delve into the natural health products that you can call on to address problems. These chapters won't be an attempt to present an encyclopedia of medical problems, an all-encompassing review of cutting-edge testing science or a comprehensive catalogue of natural health remedies. However, I do want to offer some idea of the breadth and depth of natural and alternative medicine, and share my knowledge of its products and procedures, most of which will be of use to every individual who's willing to try them.

Let's get under way, then, by focusing on those areas—seven broad categories of health concerns—that patients, readers and audiences regularly bring to my attention. As we tour through these categories, we're going to stop here and there to consider that we may not always be as healthy as we think we are—or as we might easily be. We'll also sample from the vast array of testing that is now available to laypersons—either directly or through their health practitioners.

I'd like to emphasize that we're not going to spend a lot of time on the common testing that determines your current state of health—blood pressure, hip-waist measurement ratio, cholesterol and so on—because your doctor will already have such metrics on file. We'll be talking instead about testing for subclinical deficiencies—the kind that hide under the radar and cause symptoms but not full-blown disease. We'll be talking about something called "predictive genomics"—testing that looks under the hood of your DNA to give you an idea of what you should do *now* in order to prevent future disease. We're going to be talking about "functional testing" too, a subject I touched on in *The Antioxidant Prescription* and am excited to share with you. Functional testing asks questions like "*How well* is my immune system working?" as opposed to "Do I have an infection?" or "Is there something going on in me that shouldn't be?" I'll be basing this chapter on testing models that travel well outside the conventional standard, outside the bare minimum "Let's-make-sure-Mr.-Jones-won't-die-tomorrow" mentality. Testing for these sorts of high or low but "normal" results requires that you be tested fairly regularly and know what the "normal" versus the "optimal" ranges for those tests are. And testing of this sort requires you to be astute, with a keen interest in your health.

I can't even pretend to be presenting a comprehensive catalogue of testing. It would be daunting, overwhelming and, frankly, nearly impossible to include everything I'd like to about how to best assess your current state of health. The so-called executive medical practices—MedCan, Cleveland Clinic, Medisys, Mayo, etc.—all have great (and yet still somewhat incomplete) models, consisting of dozens of tests to help determine the state of health of a person who can afford thousands of dollars in testing beyond what public or private insurers cover. That may be the best that money can buy, but we'll be looking at what intelligent interest, reasonable concern and ordinary finances can obtain for you as an individual.

1. THEY'VE GOT US SURROUNDED: TOXINS, INFECTIOUS AGENTS AND ALLERGENS

At first blush, you're going to wonder what I'm doing, putting hay fever, mercury poisoning and the common cold in the same category. But all these and many more afflictions have something in common: they are illnesses that arise from the interaction of external agents with our body's internal defences. These agents are all around us and often inside us. Some we have deliberately or unwittingly introduced into our environment. Others have been the unwelcome companions of humanity since time immemorial. Some that we've long been familiar with and considered harmless have only recently appeared in such abundance as to cause our bodies to react badly to them. In the course of our discussion, we'll look at some examples and then consider what I believe to be the most important lesson of this chapter, and perhaps the most important lesson of this book, one the Romans would have done well to consider: you can't blame the invader when your defences are weak.

TOXINS

It is becoming more apparent that what doesn't hurt you now may kill you later. A few decades ago, you rarely heard the term "chemical toxin." If something could poison you, it was called "poison." Everyone knew what poisons were: products labelled with a skull and crossbones, such as the bleach in your laundry room. You knew they were dangerous and you kept them away from the kids. Today we're less concerned with "poisons" and more concerned with "toxins"—a word with a subtly different meaning and a word on everyone's lips. Indeed, toxins are often literally on our lips. Most of us are aware that pre-1980s paint may contain lead that you have to be careful about removing, but we aren't aware that many of us are applying it to our lips every day in the form of lipsick. The reality is with no required safety testing, cosmetics companies can use almost any chemical they choose, regardless of risks. Damaging chemicals—oxybenzone, ethylhexyl methoxycinnamate, retinyl palmitate and a whole lot more—crop up in medicine cabinets and handbags. We can't trust claims like "dermatologist-tested," "natural" or "organic" because there's no one to verify these claims when it comes to cosmetics. If we care about our health, we're expected to become biochemists overnight to be able to read and understand the ingredients labels.

Plastics—another example of potential toxins—are but one group of the chemical-emitting products in our houses that we come into contact with every day. Man-made chemicals can contribute to fatigue, chronic illness, genetic mutation and even cancer. While it's impossible to avoid these chemicals altogether, it only makes sense to lower our exposure whenever we can.

The most common sources of toxic exposure are encountered in the course of our everyday activities. Breathing, eating and drinking—all necessary for life—happen to be the top three ways toxins enter our systems. Many environmental toxins are stored in fat cells and increase in the body over one's

To watch a clip about the toxins in the home, scan the QR barcode above into your smart device or enter the following link into your browser: http://bit.ly/SR9ZmO

lifetime, disrupting the immune, nervous and hormone systems. A toxic burden can be the underlying source of many immune-related or other chronic illnesses and you may be surprised to learn that these toxins can be passed on to future generations, increasing the risk of childhood diseases such as leukemia and other cancers, asthma, autism and ADD/ADHD, to name a few.

Evaluating Your Toxin Exposure

Testing for environmental toxins should be the first step to help you get back on the road to wellness. Following are the most likely places you'll find toxins in your day-to-day life.

Your dresser top, your children's bedroom and the medicine cabinet

Phthalates and parabens can be found in children's toys, cosmetics, cleaning products, air fresheners, perfumes, furniture, vinyl flooring, plastic food containers and medical products. Phthalates and parabens are often classified as "xenoestrogens," foreign compounds in the body that bind specifically to estrogen receptors and function as hormone mimickers and not surprisingly as hormone disruptors. Researchers have studied the phthalate and paraben concentrations in everyday products, but you may have yourself tested to determine how much of the insidious chemicals you personally contain.

Your pantry and kitchen cupboards

Bisphenol-A (BPA) is still a common ingredient in plastics associated with food storage, regardless of warnings issued years ago that it contributes to cancer. Sure, they replaced most of the baby bottles that contained it, but nearly every canned food still has a liner within it that contains BPA. I was upset recently to discover that the holding tank on my reverse osmosis water filter had a lining within it containing BPA. Testing yourself for bisphenol-A might be a good idea and can also help identify exposure to other common hormone disruptors like triclosan (an antimicrobial found in many hand soaps, hand sanitizers, some toothpaste and other cosmetics) and 4-nonylphenol (found in industrial detergents, foaming agents, dispersants and emulsifiers).

Your water supply

Chlorinated pesticides have been used in agriculture worldwide since World War II, and as insecticides to exterminate mosquitoes, termites and fire ants. Dichlorodiphenyltrichloroethane (DDT) is the best-known organochlorine insecticide. Although they're now largely banned in Canada and the United States, they continue to contaminate soil and groundwater and through these routes can ultimately enter our nervous systems. Infants can be exposed through breastfeeding.

The Center of Disease Control (CDC) lists normal reference ranges for chlorinated pesticides including DDT in human blood that has been documented to cause adverse health problems. You can have yourself tested for chlorinated pesticides to help identify when or if you may have been exposed to certain pesticides and insecticides, and how high a body burden of chlorinated pesticides you are carrying. Levels are given both in parts per billion (PPB) and as lipid-adjusted amounts so your clinician can best estimate the total body burden of DDT or any other chlorinated pesticide. Chlorinated pesticides have an affinity for fat-rich tissues, and are stored in various organs—shockingly, they have been identified in over 98 percent of all persons studied. These toxins "bioaccumulate" in our bodies, increasing our toxic burden over time, and are powerful mitochondrial toxins. Mitochondria are the powerhouses of every cell in your body that work to create the biological currency of energy we know as ATP. Pesticides disturb the natural process of mitochondrial energy production. They may also be the root cause of many chronic illnesses, including Parkinson's.

Your refrigerator

PCBs once were used as lubricants and coolants in transformers, capacitors and electronic equipment because of a high resistance to heat. They were banned in the late 1970s when studies showed they contributed to severe acne, rashes, eye irritation, liver damage, weakened immune system, allergies, obesity, chronic fatigue, certain cancers and developmental disorders. But due to the stability of the compounds, they do not break down in the environment and gradually accumulate in the fatty tissues of animals and humans. They travel up the food chain in fish, fatty meats and dairy products. They also show up in breast milk.

In the vegetable crisper

Organophosphates have found widespread application since the 1950s as pesticides and most exposure occurs from ingestion through our food supply. Direct exposure through the skin can also occur for farmers and other people who work directly with these chemicals. Testing is important if you think you've had prolonged exposure to the organophosphates, because they've been shown to cause serious health problems such as Alzheimer's and Parkinson's disease and neurological deficits in children and babies in the womb, producing lower IQs, chronic fatigue, asthma, immune system disorders, impaired memory, disorientation, depression, irritability, flu-like symptoms and a possible increase in the risk of cancer. We want our children to eat more fruits and veggies, but a recent study found that each tenfold increase in urinary concentration of organophosphate metabolites was associated with a 55 to 72 percent increase in the odds of ADHD in children. The solution: go certified organic!

The garage

Volatile solvents such as those found in car exhaust, paints, glues, adhesives and lacquer thinners are also used in the manufacture of many consumer products: glues and adhesives, paints and paint thinners, furniture, building materials, degreasing agents, inks, pharmaceuticals and additives to gasoline and shoes. Exposure to volatile solvents is usually through inhalation of fumes or ingestion of polluted water. For those living and working in urban areas, the exposure to this class of compounds goes on twenty-four hours a day. Solvents are damaging to your bone marrow and are associated with immune disorders, chronic neurological problems and infertility. If you believe you may have had an overexposure or chronic exposure to volatile solvents, you don't need to wait until there is obvious damage to your central nervous system or chemical-driven liver and kidney damage before you ask your health care provider to help determine your levels. In particular, one solvent, benzene, has a severe toxic effect on the blood and is a known cause of cancer. Other solvents contribute to atrophy of skeletal muscles, loss of coordination, vision problems and depression of the central nervous system.

All around you

We can be exposed to so-called heavy metals—mercury, lead, arsenic and others—through a sudden poisoning incident or through long-term, low-level exposure. Heavy metal pollution from industrial processes may seem exotic, but the persistence of metals in the environment and their tendency to bioaccumulation and biomagnification is a constant factor. The warnings we hear about eating large predator fish stem from this accumulation factor. And surprisingly, many dentists continue to fill teeth with mercury, a neurotoxin.

People with excessive acute or chronic heavy metal exposure may experience fatigue, weakness, chemical sensitivity, irritability, anxiety, memory loss, insomnia, numbness and tingling in hands and feet, tremors, gastrointestinal issues and loss of appetite. If you are troubled by such symptoms, testing for individual heavy metals is always a good idea. But the symptoms of, say, mercury toxicity can be similar to those of lead or cadmium toxicity and knowing what to test for can be daunting and confusing. You can, however, be tested for porphyrins, whose chemical structures bind to heavy metals. Specific porphyrin elevations in urine may serve as functional markers that can help identify the severity of exposure to specific toxic metals.

THE INFECTIOUS AGENTS: VIRUSES, BACTERIA, FUNGI AND PARASITES

While the types of infectious agents are hugely variable, what they all have in common is their ability to invade the human body and sometimes cause disease. All infections are readily confirmed *if* you know what you're looking for. Unfortunately it's quite easy for any doctor to miss an infectious agent because there's no one single test that looks at all infectious potential. Let me suggest, however, that if you have symptoms that are strange, rare or peculiar, and you haven't been offered a satisfactory diagnosis, you may want to test for infection. What follows are a few examples of infectious agents, with special attention to some that are often overlooked or improperly tested for.

Bacteria

Bacteria constitute one of the major biological domains and are critical to sustaining life on this planet. They're also critical to the functioning of our own bodies. Bacteria are found in vast numbers on the skin, in the airways, in the mouth and in the digestive tract. Certain bacteria help digest specific types of food. Others keep infectious organisms at bay. In short, a great bunch of guys. There is no need to kill 99.9 percent of them after all—in fact we *may* be doing more harm than good.

A few types of bacteria, alas, have gone bad in human terms and are major causes of disease and suffering. They may invade the body through the skin or orifices, begin to multiply and go on to harm the body. That's a bacterial infection, and it can lead to serious complications or death. However, if such infections are diagnosed and treated quickly, most patients today experience a complete recovery and enjoy an even more robust immunity thereafter.

During the twentieth century, one of the great advances in medicine was the development of antibiotics, which are often lifesaving. However, many doctors, scientists and epidemiologists have grown concerned about bacteria that have developed resistance to antibiotics. One of the most recent examples of these new antibiotic-resistant "bugs" is methicillin-resistant *Staphylococcus aureus* (or MRSA), which can flourish in hospitals despite our best antibiotics. Even more recently the World Health Organization reported the dangerous sexually transmitted disease gonorrhea, which infects millions of people each year, is growing resistant to drugs and could soon become untreatable.

Lyme disease. Lyme disease is a worldwide infectious disease caused by a spirochete spiral bacteria, *Borrelia burgdorferi*, that is transmitted to people by tiny insects called ticks. They are dangerous, double-membraned bacteria, most of which are long and helically coiled, that is, spiral-shaped. Ticks that carry them are found across North America, and people walking through woodlands and brushy areas may pick up a tick without knowing it. The tick, the size of a poppy seed, burrows into the skin and remains for hours or days while it engorges itself with blood. If the tick is infected, the spirochete bacteria are transmitted to the bloodstream of the person.

Early recognition is key. If you're in a known tick-infested area, carefully inspect your skin for ticks and if you find one, immediately report to a hospital emergency room if possible for proper removal, diagnosis and treatment. In some patients who are actually infected (fewer than 40 percent), a characteristic red bull's-eye rash may develop at the site of the bite. The rash may appear within days to weeks after the bite, but could be hidden in the hairline or underarms. For that reason, you should preserve an extracted tick in a moist tissue and see your physician immediately. Many jurisdictions have set up labs to test ticks for disease, so consider keeping them if you find one on your body. A simple blood test for antibodies to the bacterium is the preferred test for the diagnosis. However, if a person has central nervous system symptoms, such as meningitis, then IgM, IgG and Western blot testing may sometimes be performed on cerebral spinal fluid. A polymerase chain reaction (PCR) test may also be performed on a sample because it is a more sensitive way of detecting Lyme disease. This method looks for the genetic material (DNA) of *B. burgdorferi* in samples such as joint fluid (synovial fluid). If the result from PCR testing is positive, then it indicates infection. But if the PCR test result is negative, then there *may* be no infection present *or* the levels of DNA may be too low to detect.

What you need to know is that Lyme disease (especially in a chronic or "late" state and when left untreated and undiagnosed) is a great imitator because so many of the signs and symptoms are indistinguishable from those of other diseases. Co-infections such as babesiosis (caused by parasites) that can be transmitted *with* Lyme have symptoms that can easily be mistaken for those of other ailments such as chronic fatigue syndrome and fibromyalgia. Ticks can unfortunately carry a lot of disease.

Lyme disease is serious, so if you think you may have it, get comprehensive testing, and don't rely on the results of any one test alone. If possible, see a doctor who takes a special interest in Lyme disease.

Consider sending samples to these laboratories for a more comprehensive workup:

www.igenex.com
www.neurorelief.com

H. pylori. If you experience chronic reflux, heartburn, gas and bloating or if you have more serious symptoms of gastrointestinal pain, unexplained weight loss, and nausea or vomiting you should be screened for the bacteria *Helicobacter pylori.*

A positive *H. pylori* blood antibody test, a stool antigen test or a positive breath test indicates you have been infected with this organism. Scientific studies have now established that *H. pylori* can cause peptic ulcers and is a strong risk factor for certain types of stomach cancer. A negative test may mean that you are not infected. However, the gold standard is to have a tissue biopsy of the stomach to more conclusively rule out a current infection.

Viruses

Viruses are organisms so primitive that they're referred to as viral particles and cannot even reproduce except inside the cells of living organisms. Nonetheless they account for much human misery. They cause disease by destroying or damaging the cells they infect, damaging the body's immune system, changing the genetic material of cells and causing inflammation that damages joints and organs. We can attribute to viruses such diseases as AIDS, caused by the human immunodeficiency virus (HIV), cold sores, chicken pox, measles, influenza and some types of cancer. Both bacteria and viruses are detectable, but whereas bacteria-caused diseases may be entirely curable, viruses are usually not more than treatable; that is, only the symptoms can be relieved.

Several types of tests may be used to check for viruses:

- *Antibody test.* Antibodies are proteins created by the body's immune system to fight a specific viral infection. They attach to a cell infected by the virus and cause the virus to be destroyed. This test generally uses a blood sample and looks for antibodies to a specific viral infection. If the antibody is found, this test can show whether a person was infected recently or in the past.
- *Viral antigen detection test.* Viral antigens develop on the surface of cells infected with a specific virus. A viral antigen detection test is done on a sample of tissue that might be infected. Specially tagged (with dye or a tracer) antibodies that attach to those viral antigens are mixed with the sample. The tagged antibodies can be seen by using a special light (or other method). If the tagged antibodies are attached to the cells, the cells are infected with the virus.
- Another approach to viral detection is that used for bacteria: *the culturing of viruses.* A small sample of tissue or fluid that may be infected is placed in a special cup along with cells in which the virus can grow. If the virus grows in the culture, it will cause changes in the cells that can be seen under a microscope. Electron microscopy may also be employed to visualize virus particles directly.
- A fourth approach is the *viral DNA* or *RNA detection test,* which uses a sample of tissue, blood, or perhaps spinal fluid to look for the genetic material of a specific virus. This test can determine the exact virus causing an infection.

Epstein-Barr virus. If you have been diagnosed with chronic fatigue or fibromyalgia, you may wish to check to see whether these poorly understood conditions could be the effects of Epstein-Barr virus (EBV). EBV is passed from one person to another by the sharing of food utensils, kissing, and through other means of close contact involving the saliva. When EBV enters the cell, its aim is to take control of the body's DNA and to reprogram it to make copies of itself. Alerted by the invasion, the body's immune system launches a counter-attack by sending its killer cells to destroy the virus, and in so doing produces antibodies at a high rate of speed. This complicated process may confuse viral material with your body's tissue. When the immune system makes such a mistake, antibodies created against your own body may cause the symptoms we know as fibromyalgia and chronic fatigue syndrome. A range of EBV antibody tests is available.

To watch a clip about fibromyalgia support, scan the QR barcode above into your smart device or enter the following link into your browser: http://bit.ly/MEpa3D

Cold and flu viruses. It is estimated that the average person contracts more than 150 colds during a lifetime. Anyone can get a cold, although pre-school and grade school children catch them more frequently than adolescents and adults. But the real measure of health isn't whether you come down with a cough or cold, it's how quickly you overcome it. The fact is, if you've never encountered a particular virus, you're likely to react on contact. A healthy person may develop antibodies immediately, experience no symptoms, and fight off the virus without ever knowing he or she was infected. An unhealthy person may require weeks to get better.

The common cold (a.k.a., acute viral nasopharyngitis, if you want to get technical) is a viral infection of the upper respiratory system. Colds are one of the leading causes of doctor visits and missed days from school and work. In fact, roughly 25 million school days are lost annually in North America as a result of the common cold. We spend about $2.9 billion on over-the-counter drugs in North America and another $400 million on prescription medicines annually for the symptomatic relief from colds.

Recently we've determined that much over-the-counter cough and cold medication is not only ineffective, but possibly harmful. But as we'll see, there's little reason to resort to them, because natural health products can provide effective support for coughs and colds.

What many folks don't know is that a cold or flu starts off as a viral infection but can take a turn for the worse and be complicated by a superimposed bacterial infection. Bacteria love to replicate in warm, moist, humid environments. When you are battling a virus, the mucus you produce in your upper respiratory system is a perfect breeding ground. *If* you indeed have a bacterial infection—and there are excellent ways to test for these by culturing sputum or swabbing the nose or throat—then a matched antibiotic to the diagnosed bacteria is an excellent option. Just don't forget that antibiotics do nothing for a viral infection.

To watch a clip about cold and cough support, scan the QR barcode above into your smart device or enter the following link into your browser: http://bit.ly/NQ4kK8

When it comes to the cold virus, however, I know of no laboratory test that will confirm the presence of the common cold virus. There are, however, more than 25 rapid flu tests on the market and available to your doctor. A new meta-analysis of 159 studies of the accuracy of these rapid influenza diagnostic tests (RIDTs) which was conducted by researchers at McGill University in Montreal showed that RIDTs can be used to confirm the flu but not to rule it out. The meta-analysis also showed that test accuracy is higher in children than in adults and that RIDTs are better at detecting the more common influenza A virus than influenza B.

Parasites

Parasites are organisms that live by feeding off a host organism. But we're concerned here with the sort of protozoa and worms that live off the human body, whether inside or outside the host's cells.

If you have diarrhea that lasts more than a few days or you have blood or mucus in loose stools, and especially if you have consumed unpurified water while camping or have travelled outside of North America, then testing for parasites is definitely indicated. In fact, if you have persistent immune or neurological symptoms or any set of bizarre symptoms with no logical diagnosis, then testing for ova and parasites in your stool is advisable. Not that parasites confine themselves to the digestive tract; they can set up shop anywhere in your body.

If they do decide to inhabit your GI, but no actual parasites or ova are seen in the stool, then tests for the blood antigens associated with protozoa such as *Giardia, Cryptosporidium* and *Entamoeba histolytica* can detect protein structures on the parasites and so identify an infection. These antigen tests are a good start, but they can detect only a few specific parasites and are not replacements for the complete ova and parasite stool test. Beyond these direct tests, a more comprehensive assessment of your immune system would look at your blood for certain cytokines. We'll have occasion to talk further about cytokines, the messengers of our immune systems, but for the moment I'll just say they come in different sorts. Whereas Th-1 cytokines are associated with bacterial infections and certain autoimmune disorders, Th-2 cytokines indicate allergic responses or mucosal parasitic infections.

Yeasts

Candida albicans. Candida albicans is usually a benign yeast, yeasts being classified as a form of fungus. This yeast lives in 80 percent of healthy persons, but localized outbreaks can occur on the skin, under nails or mucous membranes of the mouth, in the vagina, bronchi, or lungs. In a complex medical syndrome called chronic candidiasis, yeast syndrome, or simply candida, the overgrowth can become systemic and can cause disease.

Localized vaginal yeast infections are one of the most common reasons that women consult health-care professionals. When yeast infections cause inflammation of the vaginal canal, we refer to the condition as vaginitis. The hallmark symptom of a yeast infection is itching of the external and internal genitalia, which is often associated with a white discharge that can be thick and/or resemble cottage cheese curds. Severe infections lead to inflammation of the tissue and subsequent redness, swelling and even pinpoint bleeding.

Yeast infections are more common in women who wear nylon underwear than in those who wear cotton underwear. Additional predisposing factors for candida infection include the use of antibiotics, oral contraceptives, adrenal corticosteroids (such as prednisone), and an overload of alcohol and sugar in the diet. Underlying health conditions that may predispose someone to candida overgrowth include pregnancy, diabetes and HIV infection.

Systemic yeast is over-diagnosed in the world of alternative medicine. Although an overgrowth of candida in the gastrointestinal tract can cause fatigue, allergies, immune system malfunction, depression, chemical sensitivities and digestive disturbances, objective confirmation is required before any sort of treatment can be recommended. Conventional medical authorities acknowledge the existence of a chronic candida infection that affects the whole body and is sometimes called "chronic disseminated candidiasis." However, this universally accepted disease is both uncommon, mostly arising in those receiving chemotherapy who have profound immunosuppresion, and decidedly narrower in scope than so-called yeast syndrome.

Again, proper testing is crucial. Yeast syndrome is a condition markedly common in people with a history of long-term antibiotic use. A stool culture can provide information about the concentration of candida growth within the body. An immune response to candida by measuring blood IgG antibodies can establish current or past exposure.

ALLERGIES, SENSITIVITIES AND INTOLERANCE

If you're sniffling, sneezing and wheezing, your throat itches, your nose is running and your eyes are watery, in all likelihood you are one of the 20 percent of North Americans who are allergic to something, and that something may be in season. An allergy occurs when the body's immune system overreacts to a substance that is normally harmless, such as mould, pollen, animal dander or dust mites. It's easy to mistake allergies and hay fever symptoms for symptoms of an infection—a cold or sinusitis. But a cold usually lasts no more than ten days and often presents with thick green or yellow mucus as opposed to the clear and runny mucus of an allergy. The overall itch is often the clue that we're suffering from an allergy.

To watch a clip about allergy support, scan the QR barcode above into your smart device or enter the following link into your browser: http://bit.ly/Oinhpy

These airborne triggers are familiar to almost everyone, whether we're sufferers ourselves or not. But more complex and mysterious are our adverse reactions to the very substance that sustains us: our food. It's been long known that the consumption of certain foods can have profound effects on our individual immune systems. But I'm not speaking here of fast food, junk food, sugar, chemicals or preservatives—substances that can erode our health over a period of years. I'm speaking about food allergies and food intolerance.

Food intolerance. Also known as non-allergic food hypersensitivity, this is a distinct category of problem not to be confused with allergies. Organic dairy products may be healthy food in moderation yet more than half of the world's population will experience upset stomachs, intestinal cramps, gas or diarrhea when they ingest milk or milk products: this is lactose intolerance, the inability to effectively digest dairy, and nothing to do with immune dysfunction. Lactose, the sugar in milk, is digested by the enzyme lactase. It is estimated that 75 percent of adults worldwide show a significant—and perfectly healthy—decrease in lactase activity during adulthood. The majority of adults of Asian, African, Middle Eastern and Native American descent are lactose intolerant. In addition, 50 percent of Hispanics and about 20 percent of Caucasians do not produce sufficient lactase as adults. If a person is one of this 75 percent and drinks milk, he or she may to varying degrees experience bloating, upset stomach, loose bowels and mild to moderate forms of diarrhea.

To watch a clip about lactose intolerance, scan the QR barcode above into your smart device or enter the following link into your browser: http://bit.ly/NNIaMt

A simple test for lactose intolerance is to drink at least two eight-ounce glasses of milk on an empty stomach and note any gastrointestinal symptoms that develop in the next four hours. The test should then be repeated using several ounces of cheese (which does not contain much lactose). If symptoms result from milk but not cheese, then you probably have lactose intolerance. If symptoms occur with both milk and cheese, you may be allergic to dairy products, a quite different condition. It's rare that lactose intolerance is so severe that eating cheese causes symptoms.

Food allergies. These are something quite different. Sometimes called food sensitivities when they are relatively mild, food allergies are a notorious cause of negative effects on the body and are based on the relationship between a food and the individual immune system. Technically speaking, a food allergy is associated with the generation of immunoglobulin E (IgE) antibodies against that particular food. The symptoms may be hives, swelling or full-blown anaphylaxis. If you have a food allergy, you're probably already carrying around an EpiPen and wearing a MedicAlert bracelet.

If you experience digestive distress soon after eating but have never discerned the cause, then testing is the key to identifying whether you have a food intolerance or a food allergy. A food allergy is effectively evaluated by a blood test that looks at the immunoglobulins present in the body against specific foods. In fact, almost everyone has some allergic reaction to some food, usually the result of repeated consumption of the same food (I had a friend who ate peanut butter several times a day for forty years until it became the trigger to terrible migraines), general overconsumption or inherited susceptibility. Most people, however, do not experience intense symptoms and get by without serious problems.

An example of overconsumption in our society is the omnipresent wheat grain. A morning breakfast cereal with toast, a sandwich for lunch, crackers as a snack, pasta for dinner with cakes and cookies for dessert is not at all an uncommon diet routine in our part of the world. Given that many people have a genetic predisposition to wheat intolerance, developing a real intolerance to wheat gluten is hardly surprising. Even a mild to moderate gluten sensitivity can produce symptoms of gas, bloating, polishing of the intestine and malabsorption. Chronic inflammation to the lining of the intestine from an overactive immune system (which attacks the intestinal mucous membrane) causes the intestine to wear down ("polish") and eventually become unable to absorb nutrients. This is known as celiac disease, a genetically inherited allergy to the gluten component of wheat that affects the digestive system and especially the small intestine, and often produces more severe symptoms. Perhaps one in 117 people have full-blown celiac disease, and about 97 percent of those with the disease don't know it. If you wonder whether you or a loved one has celiac, a GP can do blood work to look at readings of anti-tissue transglutaminase antibodies, total immunoglobulins (in particular IgA) and screenings for anti-gliadin antibodies and anti-endomysial antibodies. You may be referred to a gastroenterologist for a biopsy. Alternatively, there is a widely available home blood test that allows you to do the preliminary work-up in the comfort of your own home (https://www.glutenpro.com/celiacsure.html). Report the results to your family doctor. And keep in mind that, even if you don't have celiac disease (which is what this test is looking for), you may still have a mild intolerance or sensitivity to gluten.

One way to rule in or out food intolerances and allergies is to undergo an "elimination diet" that identifies exactly what food may be causing your symptoms. The elimination diet involves entirely removing suspected food(s) from the diet for a period of time—two weeks to two months—and waiting to determine whether symptoms resolve. Then you purposely reintroduce items one at a time into the diet while leaving three days between each reintroduced food as you chart symptoms and responses.

If it's irritable bowel syndrome (IBS) you suffer from and you think dairy in particular is something you want to rule in or out, ask your doctor to conduct a hydrogen breath test (HBT). An HBT can also help determine whether or not you have bacterial imbalance in the gut.

A skin *allergy* test determines fixed or immediate responses to food allergies. A simple test your doctor can do involves scratching your arm and/or back with suspected allergens and then analyzing the welts left behind for their intensity.

Food *sensitivity* testing (very different than intolerance or allergy), however, is done when certain symptoms develop, or preexisting conditions become worse. Examples of such symptoms include acne, anxiety, arthritis, asthma, attention deficit disorder, autism, chronic diarrhea, chronic fatigue, constipation, depression, diabetes, high blood pressure, hyperactivity disorder, irritable bowel syndrome, muscle pain, obesity, panic attacks, sinusitis and weight imbalance. Again, we're not talking about the difference between good foods and bad foods when we're talking about these immune responses. An IgG reaction can be triggered by such wholesome foods as organic chicken, broccoli or spinach. True, the reactions that sensitivities provoke are not as severe as allergies, but they can nonetheless damage your health through inflammation and the sort of symptoms I've just listed.

Testing your blood is the first step in the process to help identify the foods that may be causing symptoms. Professional laboratories use the microarray-based test that can detect IgG antibodies to more than two hundred different foods. A blood test is a good way to reveal hidden food sensitivity in these circumstances. Another interesting investigation method employs electro-dermal testing—a discovery made by Dr. Reinhold Voll in the 1950s—that gauges electrical skin resistance and provides information about your chi (or energy pathways) in a non-invasive way. A well-respected and scientifically proven testing protocol called the enzyme-linked immunosorbant assay provides a useful measurement of the concentration of the antigen (the food in question) and the antibody (your immune response), thereby exposing the specific food intolerance. These factors are determined by an immune reaction governed by a molecular component of the immune system called immunoglobulin gamma (IgG). Based on test results, patients can then work with their health professionals, using an elimination diet to determine which foods should be eliminated or reduced from their diets. The old saying "one man's meat is another man's poison" really is true. No test is 100 percent accurate, and food allergy testing is no exception. Although results are highly reproducible, you can expect a few false positives and negatives (e.g., cashews may show up as sensitive, but on a subsequent test, they don't. Pepper spice may not show up as positive, but a subsequent test might suggest a low-grade response).

To watch a clip about what makes your allergies worse, scan the QR barcode above into your smart device or enter the following link into your browser: http://bit.ly/NO9OIf

In many cases, eliminating these sensitivity triggers from your diet may be enough to relax an overexcited immune system and you may find yourself symptom free. I've personally witnessed hundreds of cases of eczema, psoriasis, migraine headaches, fibromyalgia, irritable bowel syndrome and panic attacks that quite literally disappear once food intolerances were tested for, discovered and removed.

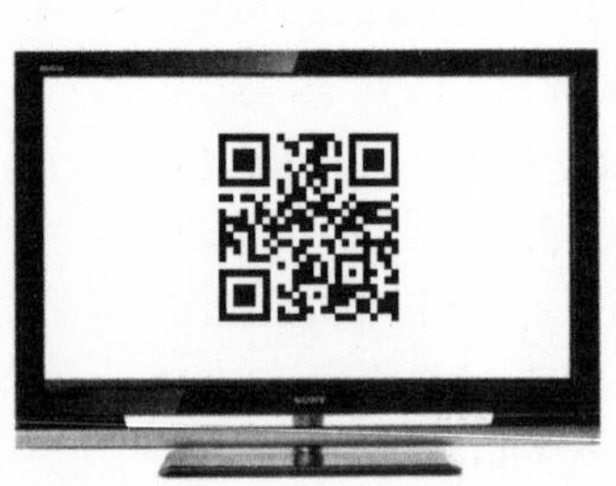

To watch a clip about psoriasis and eczema support, scan the QR barcode above into your smart device or enter the following link into your browser: http://bit.ly/OUSAoj

IMMUNITY: THE ENDLESS CAMPAIGN

We can't really conclude our discussion of infectious agents without taking a closer look at our immune system. The fact is—and Louis Pasteur, the man who launched the search for infectious agents, is said to have confirmed this on his deathbed—as important as infectious agents are in disease, the hosts—that's us—are even more important.

Our bodies are made up of trillions of cells, a sub-group of which flows through our bloodstream and across our mucous membranes. The role of these special cells—our white blood cells—is to protect us against infection. They are the most important part of our immune system. If we think of that immune system as an army defending us against outside invaders, we who depend on that army need to know the state of the troops.

Assessing Your Immunity Army

If your doctor thinks that you might have an infectious disease, one of the first things he or she will do is check your blood for the production of white blood cells. The test is done as part of a complete blood count (CBC), which may be ordered for a variety of reasons. An *increased* number of white blood cells can be a response to bacterial infections, inflammation, leukemia, trauma, intense exercise, stress and many other triggers. A *decreased* white blood cell count can result from chemotherapy, radiation therapy, diseases of the immune system and other causes. Counts that continue to rise or fall to abnormal levels indicate that the condition is getting worse and when counts return to normal, it typically indicates improvement.

Our white blood cell count is important because it tells us how many troops we have in our immunity army. But counting the troops doesn't give us the full story of what our immune system is actually doing. It's one thing to have thousands of soldiers, but if half of them are sleeping in and/or hungover from a night of partying, we say our "immune activity" is low. The troops aren't listening to the general in command. Fortunately, immune activity is something we can test for—one way is with a test called natural killer cell activity.

If we have an ideal number of troops, and they're all active but they're only armed with sticks and stones, they'll have a limited effect against the enemy. We want our immune army armed to the teeth with "cytotoxicity"—weaponry that's the scourge of viruses, bacteria and sundry offending agents. Fortunately, we now have the natural killer cell cytotoxicity test.

Okay, let's say you have an ideal white blood cell count, an active "army" and powerful weaponry with the latest technology. But wait—what if communications are down? What if the officers in command can't communicate and the immunity army doesn't know if it should attack, what to attack, or for how long? Ah, but that's where the cytokines come in. These are the busy runners between immunity command and the immunity troops. Depending on which white blood cells are to be called into action during an immune response, specific cytokines flood the field to carry instructions that shift the balance of an immune response. This is where we need artillery, gunboats and shock troops. White blood cells need to be ready to attack!

In the absence of infection, specialized cells called macrophages, whose job it is to gobble up invaders, inhibit the activation and development of immune cells. In this case the orders are to generally stand down. Otherwise, it is their nature to keep on gobbling. Early in an infection, immune system officers call out the non-coms to ready their troops, and part of the immune system is alerted as though air raid sirens have gone off. Then, depending on the threat level, all hell can break loose as orders are released to the major pro-inflammatory immune cells. Once an infection takes hold, the generals in command instruct the special forces (previously holding rank in a watch-and-wait pattern) to stand down. Now the infantry is dispatched, tanks roll out, and air strikes are launched. At this point, the immune response is to seek and destroy.

Your Genetic Destiny

In the end, an effective immunity army isn't something you can just buy. It's to some degree something you're born with—a gift from Mom and Dad with help from your grandmas and grandpas on each side.

Now comes the really interesting news. Recent discoveries are teaching us that if we can't change our genes, we *can* at least modify the "expression" of those genes, that is, how the genes actively influence the body's functioning. Researchers have developed testing that allows us to evaluate variations to genes, variations called single nucleotide polymorphisms (SNPs)—polymorphism being another word for mutation. Certain genes are in charge of the health of the immune system and these to some degree control inflammation and affect immune system balance and function. SNPs in these genes can trigger potential defects in our immune defences. Ultimately, such mutations can create chronic, overactive inflammatory responses and immune system breakdown.

In what follows, I'm going to talk about testing certain genes to reveal SNPs. Testing of this kind can give us insight into what we must do to prevent these modified genes from acting up prematurely. If we know which of our genes have mutated, we can give attention to prevention in the areas they affect; we can alter our diet, get better control of our stress, exercise more or supplement appropriately and put years on our lives. Experts have coined the term "nutrigenomics" to describe the impact nutrition can have on our genes. This is truly a whole new world of applied genetics.

IL-1ß (or interleukin-1 beta) is produced by white blood cells and acts as an inflammatory-response-producing cytokine that among other things can inhibit acid secretion in the stomach and stimulate bone loss. Mutations on the gene that controls IL-1ß can lead to increased inflammation suppress hydrochloric acid secretion in the stomach and increase susceptibility to *Helicobacter pylori* infection and gastritis and gastric cancer in *H. pylori*–infected individuals. Paradoxically, the mutation may provide some slight protection against breast and lung cancer. If someone with this genetic glitch also had an *H. pylori* infection, eradication of the infection and mucous membrane repair are essential due to the increased risk of gastric cancer. Once the damage has been repaired, regular betaine hydrochloride with meals may prevent a re-infection. It would be imperative to reduce alcohol consumption, avoid smoking, and increase the proportion of fruit in the diet. The individual would need to be very careful with all non-steroidal anti-inflammatory drugs (NSAIDs), such as Aspirin or Advil, which reduce gastric blood flow and actually increase IL-1ß. Production of excess IL-1ß is reduced by agents such as fish oils, L-glutamine, milkthistle (silymarin), curcumin, boswellia, ginkgo biloba and resveratrol. We'll look at these more closely in the next chapter. Any and all of them may make it into the daily supplement plan of someone with a mutation to the gene that controls IL-1ß. A bone scan would also be a good idea—especially for women who are post-menopausal.

TNF-α is tumour necrosis factor alpha, a pro-inflammatory cytokine secreted from activated white blood cells called macrophages. Macrophages play an important role in our defence against infection, but excessive TNF-α release can result in inflammatory reactions and oxidative stress. A mutation in the gene controlling TNF-α is associated with increased risk for asthma, allergic dermatitis, insulin resistance (especially in obese people), type 2 diabetes, osteoporosis, systemic lupus erythematosus and stress-induced increases in C-reactive protein. I strongly recommend stress management and low glycemic-index foods for people with gene mutations of this sort. TNF-α levels have been shown to be reduced by vitamins E and C, N-acetyl cysteine, EPA/DHA (in fish oils), curcumin, ginkgo biloba, conjugated linoleic acid, green tea, Siberian ginseng, stinging nettles, lactobacillus (a probiotic) and DHEA. Because people with the mutated versions of a gene that controls TNF-α are predisposed to chronic inflammation, C-reactive protein and erythrocyte sedimentation rate (ESR) may be warranted as a screen and to monitor the therapeutic effectiveness of any of the above supplementation.

IL-6 (known as interleukin-6). If testing determines that you have a mutation in the gene that controls for IL-6 expression, then you'll also have an excess of IL-6 production, which indicates excess inflammation in the body. Elevated IL-6 is associated with elevated triglycerides, decreased HDL ("good cholesterol") and increased fasting blood sugar. The risk of developing heart disease and adult-onset diabetes is increased substantially with this polymorphism (mutation). Since carbohydrates are the primary building block of triglyceride synthesis, a lower intake of carbohydrates and the complete elimination of simple carbohydrates is most important. This is what we mean in natural medicine when we say carbohydrates and sugar *cause* inflammation. If you have a genetic push in the direction of increased IL-6, a low-calorie, higher-protein, lower-carbohydrate, low-fat diet just makes sense for you. If on the other hand you abuse the carbs, you risk ramping up inflammation systemically. Fish oil supplementation has also been shown to lower triglyceride levels in people with this gene mutation. Chronic stress, lack of exercise and lack of sleep increase concentrations of IL-6 in all individuals, so stress reduction, more sleep and more exercise are all clearly beneficial. Supplements that improve stress levels (and adrenal function and balance) include vitamins C and B5, glycyrrhiza (licorice), and herbs such as ginseng, rhodiola, cordyceps, bacopa and ashwaganda. Both melatonin and beta-sitosterols from pine trees have been shown to decrease IL-6 production dramatically, reducing the inflammatory tendency and improving cell-mediated immunity.

At the end of this chapter, I provide links through which you can obtain this and other tests.

The immune system employs two quite different mechanisms to combat invasion and these two mechanisms must always remain in balance. Together they constitute a sort of teeter-totter that only works well if both sides are of similar weight. If the immune system is out of balance, the body is in a life-long battle; the system becomes weakened and confused and may eventually turn on itself in an autoimmune response, sending out antibodies that indiscriminately attack and damage parts of the body that were causing no trouble. Let me explain a little more about this balance.

When the body comes under attack, it uses what are known as "helper T-cells" to produce the right form of cytokines—messengers that alert the immune system. If one group or type of cytokine becomes too frequently alerted, imbalanced or dominant, chronic disease can develop.

For example, the Th1-type cytokines ("T" for "thymus" and "h" for "helper") produce inflammation to kill parasites, viruses and certain bacteria that live inside the cells. But these cytokines can also perpetuate various forms of autoimmune response including insulin-dependent diabetes mellitus.

Meanwhile, the Th2 cytokines counteract the effects of the Th1 cytokines and have an anti-inflammatory action. They also help kill pathogens that live outside the body's cells. But Th2 dominance can induce a pronounced allergic response in the body. If you suffer from IgE-mediated allergies, or asthma, you are likely to be over-producing Th2 cytokines.

Researchers working on allergies are looking at ways to drive up the Th1 response—to rebalance the system and prevent it from leaning heavily into a Th2 response—by redirecting the body into using the Th1 cytokines instead. Similarly, researchers who are working with diseases in which the Th1 response is driving the system are looking at using high-dose exposure to allergens to "kick-start" the Th2 immune response and so rebalance the system.

A set of T-helper cells—Th17 cells—has been newly identified. These are found where the body's internal and external environments interact—the skin, for example, and the lining of the intestinal tract. They attack bacteria on those surfaces, but do so with a lot of pro-inflammatory action. Th17 cells are thought to be implicated in Crohn's disease (an inflammation of the small intestine), ulcerative colitis (inflammation of the large intestine) and psoriasis (inflammation of the skin). It seems deficiency of probiotics (good bacteria) has a lot to do with an imbalance of Th17. With the advances in testing science, we can now assess the levels of Th1/Th2/Th17 *and* the genetics that control them.

2. THE DIGESTIVE SYSTEM

DIGESTION AND INDIGESTION

Believe it or not, it takes about a third of our daily energy output to drive our digestive system. That's an enormous amount when you consider that the other two-thirds must be shared by all of the body's other activities: maintaining body temperature, keeping our brains busy and regulating the action of our muscles. When things go wrong with our digestion, diseases such as gastroesophageal reflux disease (GERD),

To watch a clip about digestion support, scan the QR barcode above into your smart device or enter the following link into your browser: http://bit.ly/OcbsCW

irritable bowel syndrome (IBS), inflammatory bowel disease and colorectal cancer can arise. Less obviously, disorders of the skin, allergies, asthma and autoimmune dysfunctions can originate in gastrointestinal disturbances. The connection is becoming apparent with new research focused on things like the balancing act between Th1 and Th2 and particularly Th17. Before we look at how we can assess the health of our digestive organs, let's stop by a few of the problems that can afflict this critical system.

Plain Old Indigestion

Whether it's constipation, diarrhea, irritable bowel syndrome, acid indigestion, gas or bloating, every one of us occasionally experiences some form of indigestion. You've probably had some sort of mild encounter in the last few weeks.

In some cases, such as the lactose intolerance and celiac disease we looked at in the last section, symptoms of indigestion are due to a specific cause that requires specific treatment. Sometimes symptoms associated with indigestion are caused by diseases unrelated to the gastrointestinal tract. Ovarian cancer, for example, may cause a sensation of bloating and the symptoms of heartburn may sometimes be a precursor to a heart attack. So before anything else, let's say that anyone with persistent symptoms of indigestion should be properly diagnosed by a health-care professional before assuming that what they are experiencing is a simple case of "indigestion."

To watch a clip about colic support, scan the QR barcode above into your smart device or enter the following link into your browser: http://bit.ly/PBrDuL

One of the most common sorts of indigestion is heartburn, that burning sensation in the chest that may occur when the sphincter between the esophagus and the stomach is not functioning properly. A related cause of heartburn is diaphragmatic or hiatus sliding hernia, in which a small portion of the stomach protrudes through the diaphragm into the chest cavity. Even babies may not be immune, as many believe that colic is the infant's version of indigestion.

Bowel Distress

Colon health and regularity in bowel movements is a cornerstone of overall health. Many health experts believe that constipation or diarrhea are signs that the body is dealing with toxins that it has been unable to rid itself of fast enough. It has been reported that 12 percent of people worldwide suffer from constipation. Generally speaking, having a bowel movement fewer than three times a week is not healthy. Common causes of constipation include prescription medications, hormonal changes, poor bowel habits, diet, dehydration, magnesium deficiency, lack of exercise, laxatives, diseases such as colon cancer and irritable bowel syndrome (IBS) and stress.

Constipation that comes on suddenly should be evaluated by a doctor to make sure no serious disease is involved. Otherwise, natural health products should be your first response to change in normal bowel habits that is characterized by a decrease in frequency and the passage of hard, dry stools.

To watch a clip about intestinal support, scan the QR barcode above into your smart device or enter the following link into your browser: http://bit.ly/MEsP1f

Crohn's disease and ulcerative colitis have similar symptoms and are often difficult to distinguish. They are both chronic inflammatory bowel diseases (IBD) that most commonly affect the small intestine and/or colon. An estimated half million North Americans have Crohn's disease. It causes painful swelling that often results in diarrhea or frequent loose watery stools. The cause of Crohn's disease remains unknown but current research suggests that the inflammation in Crohn's disease involves a complex interaction of factors including heredity, the immune system and antigens in the environment. Blood in the stool, nocturnal bowel motions and weight loss accompanied by bowel habit changes are all red flags of more serious disease.

Invisible Leaks

Many alternative, integrative and natural health practitioners now believe that "leaky gut syndrome" or more palatably "permeable bowel syndrome" is a condition in which the intestinal walls allow food particles to pass into the bloodstream that should not be able to do so. Our digestive tract—primarily the upper segment of the small intestine—is meant to be permeable but only selectively so. Once *selective* permeability is compromised so that larger than acceptable food particles get through, the immune system considers them to be foreign invaders and the attack begins.

Our digestive system is a tube about thirty feet long running through our bodies from mouth to anus. But it is much more than that. Consider the atmosphere surrounding the earth and its protective role for our environment. Earth's atmosphere provides a protective barrier to support and sustain an abundant variety of life, and key to this is the critical balance of the different gases that provide the earth with important filter-like protection, enabling it to support the life of its 30 million different species of inhabitants. The intestine provides a similar protective barrier. The intestinal wall is coated with thousands of different species of microorganisms, both "good" and "bad" (from our perspective) bacteria, numbering in the billions. That bacterial lining is like Earth's protective atmosphere. Scientists have discovered that more bacteria reside in our gut than there are cells in the body. This rich, protective coating of microorganisms acts in concert with the physical barrier provided by the cells lining the intestinal tract and other factors to provide the body with important filter-like protection. Damaging substances—disease-causing bacteria, toxins, chemicals and wastes—are filtered out and eliminated. Simultaneously, the critical nutrients needed for the myriad of essential reactions that support life—small sugars, fats, proteins and water—are absorbed into circulation and made available to the billions of cells. At the same time, damaging substances from unhealthy bacteria, incompletely digested food, toxins or chemicals are largely prevented from being absorbed and transported throughout the body.

Unfortunately, just as in the case of our planetary atomosphere, humans' bad habits have promoted imbalance in the intestinal tract. Just as pollutants such as CFCs have punched holes in our ozone shield, dietary behaviours have contributed to an imbalance of intestinal protective factors in an alarming percentage of the population. These bad habits include widespread consumption of a diet high in refined simple sugars and deficient foods, excess alcohol, antacids, non-steroidal anti-inflammatory pain relievers, and excessive antibiotics. This tips the intestinal balance towards the overgrowth of unhealthy bacteria and a proliferation of yeast and fungal organisms, an imbalance that is also associated with chronic intestinal dysfunction.

Liver Disorders

I'm grouping the liver here with the digestive organs because that's most often how we think of it. But the liver is the second-largest organ in the body (after the skin) and plays a comparably large and complex role—many roles in fact. It processes nutrients, manufactures bile to help digest fats, synthesizes important proteins, regulates blood clotting and breaks down potentially toxic substances into harmless ones that the body can use or

To watch a clip about liver support, scan the QR barcode above into your smart device or enter the following link into your browser: http://bit.ly/NH6Zr2

excrete. Among its special features, the liver is better able to regenerate itself than any other organ, with healthy cells taking over the function of damaged cells, either indefinitely or until the damage is repaired.

Due to the complexity of the liver, there are many types of liver disease, but regardless of the type, damage to the liver is likely to progress in a similar way. Liver cells die and fat cells and dysfunctional cells take their place until new and functional liver cells replace them. If demand for new cells exceeds the available supply, liver disease ensues. Viruses such as hepatitis B and C cause much of the known liver disease worldwide. In fact, more than a million North Americans have chronic hepatitis. Other types of liver damage can be the result of drugs (such as the overuse of the popular over-the-counter pain medication acetaminophen), poisons or drinking too much alcohol over an extended period of time.

The Peptic Ulcer

There are many types of ulcers, some more serious than others. Most of us, when we speak of ulcers, are referring to the most common sort, peptic ulcers, erosions of the mucosal lining of the digestive tract that are bigger than about half a centimetre. Peptic ulcers are classified as either duodenal ulcers in the duodenum (the first part of the small intestine, just below the stomach) or gastric ulcers in the stomach itself.

Peptic ulcers can cause serious discomfort and damage to the digestive system if left untreated. Common symptoms include weight loss, bloating, belching, nausea and pain in the upper abdomen, though occasionally they are painless. Untreated, peptic ulcers often bleed and may cause a sharp burning pain in the area of the stomach or just below it. If your doctor suspects an ulcer, he or she will want to investigate whether it is associated with *Helicobacter pylori*, a stubborn bacterial infection that requires specific treatment. *H. pylori* is now believed to be the main causative factor in peptic ulcers and, with this factor identified, the prevalence of this sort of ulcer is declining. However, longer-term use of NSAIDs such as aspirin and ibuprofen have also been shown to contribute to the development of ulcers. Stress too appears to be a real factor.

To watch a clip about ulcer support, scan the QR barcode above into your smart device or enter the following link into your browser: http://bit.ly/NsjmtX

The Gall and Its Stones

The gallbladder is a small sac-like organ that concentrates bile produced by the liver for the digestion of fat. Unfortunately, the gallbladder is most famous for its production of gallstones, concretions of bile that develop inside the gallbladder. Although small in size, gallstones can cause big discomfort. Gallstone attacks can cause extreme pain in the upper-right quarter of the abdomen, often extending to the back and accompanied by nausea and vomiting. Gallstones are commonly associated with bile that contains excessive cholesterol, a deficiency of other substances in bile (bile acids and lecithin) or a combination of these factors.

To watch a clip about gallstone support, scan the QR barcode above into your smart device or enter the following link into your browser: http://bit.ly/MXcRtb

The Kidneys and Their Stones

And while we're on the subject of stones, and even though the kidneys are not strictly speaking part of the digestive system, let me mention kidney stones. If you've ever suffered from this condition, you'll know that it can cause severe back or flank pain that may radiate down to the groin region, sometimes accompanied by gastrointestinal symptoms, chills, fever and blood in the urine. Nothing you'll forget too soon.

Kidney stones are hard masses that grow from crystals formed within the kidneys. Most are composed of calcium oxalate but approximately one stone in three is made of something other than calcium oxalate and one in five contains little calcium in any form. If you have a history of kidney stone formation, you should talk with your doctor to learn what type of stones you have. That information may have a real bearing on your health, as we'll see in the next chapter.

TESTING OUR DIGESTIVE SYSTEM

So those are some of the ways our digestion can go wrong. But what should we actually be testing?

The functional status of the organs that digest and assimilate may not be on every doctor's radar but there are real consequences if your digestive system fails to carry out its tasks. There may be any number of potential causes of such failures but it's always wise to consider this: many problems originating in the gut may be related to nutritional deficiency.

I've already mentioned the hundreds of bacteria, protozoa and fungi that occupy every nook and cranny of the digestive tract. These microbes—both the pathogenic and non-pathogenic—have one thing in common: *they're supposed to be there.* It's when they become disproportionate, with too many of the pathogenic or unfriendly kind, that we have a problem.

Digestive secretions from the stomach, liver and pancreas are largely produced in response to food in the tract, and vary according to the amount and type of food present. The enteric nervous system, which is largely independent of the brain, regulates the digestion and absorption activities in concert with the immune system and independent signals from our senses. Our health is at risk if the supply of any of these secretions becomes deficient, or if the organs produce too much.

Invasive procedures for observation or specimen retrieval can be highly informative and are generally considered the gold standard of digestive testing. However, they can only be performed by specialists and are often expensive, uncomfortable, and frankly carry significant risk. If you're experiencing digestive symptoms and have not been referred to a specialist, there are many helpful and revealing tests available that are typically ignored by conventional practice.

Assessing Your Stomach Acid Balance

Problems of intestinal absorption—a major cause of indigestion—are often due to inadequate secretion of the stomach enzyme hydrochloric acid (HCl), especially in people over fifty years of age. In fact, symptoms of *inadequate* stomach acid—a burning sensation in the upper abdomen at mealtime—are similar to those of *excess* acid and one is frequently confused for the other. If you have indigestion and would like to determine whether it's due to over- or under-production of the stomach enzyme HCl, you might consider having the accurate Heidelberg capsule test. This decidedly high-tech procedure requires you to swallow a tiny plastic-encapsulated pH probe small enough to safely pass through the GI tract. It contains a miniature radio transmitter that continuously measures gastrointestinal pH and transmits the data to a waistband antenna connected to a bedside receiver. It can be difficult to locate a practitioner who performs this test, so you yourself can perform a self-test that, while less accurate, is more accessible to the average person. It is performed over a period of three days under the supervision of a GI specialist. Do not proceed with this test if you have a known ulcer or inflammatory bowel disease.

On the first day of the test, upon arising and thirty minutes before breakfast, your practitioner may advise you to take 10 grains (650 mg) of betaine HCl in a capsule form. If any discomfort, nausea or burning occurs, you will immediately discontinue the betaine HCl and inform your practitioner. People experience the discomfort differently. It is often described as an intense warmth and heaviness, like taking an ounce or two of hard liquor on an empty stomach. If no discomfort occurs, on the second day your practitioner may advise you to take two capsules instead of one. If there is any discomfort with two capsules, then a longer-term dose of one capsule with each meal will be recommended. If there is no discomfort, on the third day, you will be advised to take three capsules. If there is any discomfort with three capsules, then the long-term dose recommended is often two capsules with each meal. If there is no discomfort, then the dose will be three capsules with each meal.

Once the dose is determined, that amount is usually taken at the beginning of each meal until eventually the prescribed dose may cause discomfort. In consulting the prescribing practitioner, the typical advice is to reduce the dose by one and continue—until the point where discomfort may occur again. At that point, the treatment is typically discontinued indefinitely.

People should not take betaine hydrochloric acid capsules or tablets if they have an ulcer anywhere in the GI tract or are taking anything that might irritate the stomach lining such as aspirin, indomethacin, Bufferin, Anacin, butazolidine, cortisone or Midol. Hydrochloric acid capsules or tablets should not be chewed or opened and mixed into liquid as the acid will damage teeth and can burn the throat.

Assessing Other Digestive Functions

Digestion consists of chewing, enzyme and stomach acid production, pancreatic activity, liver bile flow, the activation of microscopic absorption areas of your pipes (called the brush border) to absorb efficiently and not "leak," and, finally, effective elimination. All of these happen in the digestive system and all can be assessed to determine your digestive health using available testing—but testing that your doctor is likely unfamiliar with.

A good preliminary assessment tool to use that determines whether the digestive system is in good order or compromised is called the urine indican test. Indican is a by-product of putrefaction, the *anaerobic* bacterial decomposition of proteins in the intestine. Putrefaction is not a healthy way for your body to deal with proteins. An elevated urinary indican is associated with such pathologic conditions as low stomach acid production, poor peristaltic movement (the "waves" that move food through the bowel) and poor production of digestive bile secretions from the gallbladder and liver. The urine indican test is generally a good indicator for the poor breakdown of proteins accompanied by the gastrointestinal permeability we call "leaky gut syndrome."

To watch a clip about leaky gut support, scan the QR barcode above into your smart device or enter the following link into your browser: http://bit.ly/MjCtBS

Digestive functions can also be assessed by submitting a stool test to a qualified laboratory to check for chemical markers that can indicate imbalances. Decreased pancreatic function is linked to gallstones, diabetes, osteoporosis and autoimmune diseases. Abnormal levels of short chain fatty acids may indicate alterations in gut flora, insufficient dietary fibre, altered transit time and small bowel bacteria overgrowth. Bile acids on the other hand play an important role in fat breakdown and absorption and high levels of some bile acids are associated with increased toxin buildup, increased risk of gallstones and gastro-intestinal cancers. Elevations of calprotectin and/or eosinophil protein X can signify mild, moderate or severe inflammation within the GI tract which is associated with infection (bacterial, viral or parasitic), food allergies, NSAID enteropathy (inflammation from overuse of aspirin or ibuprofen), IBD and even cancer.

Upwards of 80 percent of your immune system, known as gut-associated lymphatic tissue or GALT, is found in your gut. Much of GALT's effectiveness relies on the amount and activity of the beneficial flora (bacteria) that flourish there. Keeping these levels healthy is imperative for your overall health. If you think you have digestive problems, it's important to have tests performed to measure the beneficial flora such as lactobacillus and bifidobacterium, and of course any bacteria that are strictly pathogenic as well as other, potentially pathogenic bacteria and yeast.

Genomic Tests: Decoding the Warnings

We've already discussed the fact that we can't change our genes but we now know we can modify their expression. That's why it makes sense to evaluate our genetic variations: SNPs (single nucleotide polymorphisms), alleles and CNVs (copy number variations) that are all the result of natural mutations. If we consider the analogy that our genome is like a 23-volume encyclopedia, SNPs are variations scattered through all volumes that constitute a change of a single letter in a word, while alleles are whole word changes, and CNVs are deletions or additions of large amounts of genetic material comparable to whole paragraphs or pages. It is now known that some of these SNPs and CNVs are associated with increased risk of impaired detoxification capacity, especially if we're exposed to environmental toxins. Testing SNPs and CNVs can also identify a potential susceptibility to adverse drug reactions. This is called pharmacogenomics. With this unprecedented access to information about our genetic selves, we can give greater attention to prevention of conditions that would formerly have been seen as inevitable. We might alter our diet, get better control of our stress, exercise more, or supplement appropriately and thus add years on our lives. Let's look at three gene-encoded enzymes that affect the proper functioning of our liver and critically affect our capacity for digestion, nutrient dispensing and detoxification.

To watch a clip about cleansing and natural detoxification support, scan the QR barcode above into your smart device or enter the following link into your browser: http://bit.ly/PBqeEj

N-acetyl transferase (NAT) is expressed by a well-studied gene and detoxifies many environmental contaminants, including tobacco smoke and exhaust fumes. Problems with this gene may result in the slowing or acceleration of a chemical reaction called "acetylation," and either of these may be associated with increased risk of lung, colon, bladder, or head and neck cancer.

Glutathione s-transferase detoxifies many water-soluble environmental toxins, including those volatile solvents we spoke about earlier, herbicides, fungicides and heavy metals such as mercury, cadmium and lead. Defects in this detoxification activity can contribute to fatigue syndromes and many cancers.

Superoxide dismutase is a strong free radical detoxifier. Mutations on these extensively studied genes can affect this and other antioxidant enzymes. This can lead to increased free radical activity and cell damage, and may increase the risk of developing neurodegenerative disorders, heart disease and cancer.

—

There's a group of people whose ability to detoxify appears to be significantly affected by genetic glitches: those with autism spectrum disorders (ASD). Genetic detoxification impairment of course depends on the genes that govern detoxification, but some studies suggest some or all of these genes may be affected in the ASD population. Impaired detoxification in the liver results in a high level of accumulated toxins (xenobiotics) such as mercury, lead, arsenic, cadmium and aluminium. The so-called MMR vaccine controversy centres around the belief by some that mercury in the measles, mumps and rubella vaccine given in the United States (not Canada) led to an increased incidence of diagnosed autism cases. In my own view, there is a combination effect whereby an environmental trigger such as mercury, a genetic predisposition to impaired detoxification pathways and an overwhelmed immune system all contribute to the end result. When you give children with ASD supplements that aid in detoxification, they improve, some more than others. In fact, in a recent pilot trial from the Stanford University School of Medicine and Lucile Packard Children's Hospital, involving thirty-one children with ASD, found that N-acetylcysteine (NAC) may be an effective therapy for some features of autism. NAC is an antioxidant that improves our natural detoxification abilities. It seems that mainstream medicine is finally paying attention to scientifically sound interventions from the Defeat Autism Now (DAN) movement and the alternative doctors who treat autism.

If you combine genetic susceptibility with impaired liver detoxification, along with a genetic susceptibility to malformed brain cell connections, you may have the perfect storm for autism. A large international study looked at DNA mutations in genes affecting brain function and found that they appear to be a major cause of autism. The study looked for unusual DNA deletions or duplications known as "copy number variants" (CNVs) in 996 people with autism and 1,287 matched people without autism. Many of the genes in which these rare CNVs occur are linked to brain function, especially the growth and maintenance of the synapses through which brain cells communicate with each other.

Scientists have now studied many genes whose mutations (SNPs) are testable to help determine detoxification performance. We looked at a few above but there are many more—and the list is growing.

3. OF MEN AND WOMEN

SEXUALITY, GENDER AND HORMONES

Like any practitioner, I get a huge number of questions that relate to sexual function and dysfunction and to hormones. Not all hormones are directly related to sexuality, of course, so although I'm going to begin this section by talking about sexual concerns, I'll end by discussing the testing of hormonal levels in general.

To watch a clip about hormone support, scan the QR barcode above into your smart device or enter the following link into your browser: http://bit.ly/LIMbfJ

PMS

Premenstrual syndrome or PMS is a poorly understood complex of symptoms occurring a week to ten days before the start of each menstrual cycle and is believed to be triggered by changes in the levels of the hormones progesterone and estrogen. Symptoms include cramping, bloating, mood changes and breast tenderness tied to the menstrual cycle. Knowing your hormone levels by testing them and implementing lifestyle, diet and supplemental measures to

To watch a clip about menstrual support, scan the QR barcode above into your smart device or enter the following link into your browser: http://bit.ly/P5GnkG

balance them could bring the blessing of a symptom-free menstrual cycle.

Menopause

The clinical definition of menopause is that point in a woman's life when her menstrual periods stop completely and for a minimum of twelve months straight as the result of normal declines in certain hormone levels. Menopause signals the end of the ovaries releasing eggs for fertilization and generally occurs between the ages of forty-five and fifty-five, although it can occur as early as the thirties or as late as the sixties. It can also be induced by the surgical removal of both ovaries and/or by chemotherapy treatment.

There are three stages to menopause: *peri*menopause, menopause and *post*-menopause. Prior to menopause, during perimenopause, a woman may begin to experience physical and emotional signs and symptoms such as hot flashes and depression, even though she's still menstruating. The average length of perimenopause is four years, but for some women this stage may last only a few months and in others, it may continue for ten years.

To watch a clip about menopause support, scan the QR barcode above into your smart device or enter the following link into your browser: http://bit.ly/P5FI2I

Symptoms of menopause include: a change in menstruation whereby periods may be shorter or longer, lighter or heavier, with more or less time in between; hot flashes and/or night sweats; trouble sleeping; vaginal dryness; mood swings; trouble focusing; and less commonly, hair loss on the head but increased hair on the face. About 85 percent of women experiencing menopause will have hot flashes.

During post-menopause—when a year has passed since the last menstrual period—women are at a higher risk for developing osteoporosis (bone loss) and heart disease, due to the decrease in circulation of the hormone estrogen.

The Breasts

Perhaps as many as 90 percent of all women experience some symptoms such as breast pain, lumps or nipple discharge by the time they reach menopause. (A small percentage of men also experience these symptoms.) And when some concern warrants that breast tissue be examined under a microscope, some type of abnormality appears in nine out of every ten instances. Common non-cancerous breast conditions generally fall into several broad categories and include: breast pain, benign breast tumours, solitary lumps, fibrocystic changes, infections and inflammation. Some, but not all, of these benign conditions can signal an increased risk for breast cancer. To add to the baffling symptomology, most women experience physiological changes such as minor tenderness, swelling and lumpiness before or after their menstrual periods and these symptoms are absolutely normal.

Obviously, you're going to consult your doctor about unexplained breast changes. You may also be doing monthly breast self-checks already, though the benefit of these remains controversial. If not, talk to your doctor or practitioner about the techniques of self-examination. You've probably read newspaper stories about the current controversies surrounding the effectiveness of routine mammography. Your doctor should know your family and personal medical history and be able to give you sound advice on how often you should have a mammogram and whether it would be useful for you to undergo a thermography examination, which uses the body's heat rather than radiation to detect abnormalities.

To watch a clip about breast health support, scan the QR barcode above into your smart device or enter the following link into your browser: http://bit.ly/SQB4qi

The hormone estrogen breaks down into two metabolites. An excess of one can stimulate target tissues aggressively and is linked to increased risk and poorer prognosis for breast cancer, lupus and other conditions associated with "estrogen dominance." An excess of the other metabolite may increase the risk of developing conditions associated with estrogen deficiency, such as heart disease, depression and osteoporosis. A proper balance between these two products of estrogen is a key to optimal health. Since 80 percent of breast cancers are affected by estrogen, a simple twenty-four-hour urine test of estrogen balance can give clinical insight into a woman's cancer risk and the risk of many other conditions associated with estrogen dominance or deficiency. Measuring these primary estrogen metabolites allows us clinicians to develop and monitor dietary, lifestyle and hormone therapies unique to each woman's health risks.

The Prostate

Though it seems the preponderance of sexually-related afflictions fall on women, men too can struggle with health problems unique to them.

A healthy human prostate gland is about the size of a walnut. It is positioned just below the bladder and actually surrounds the urethra. Its primary function is to secrete a slightly alkaline fluid that helps neutralize the acidity of the vaginal tract, prolonging the lifespan of sperm. Male hormones produced in the testes—the androgens and in particular testosterone—stimulate the growth of the prostate.

In general, the size of the prostate remains constant after

puberty for the next thirty or more years and in some men the prostate never again increases in size. Unfortunately, most men will develop some form of non-cancerous enlargement of the prostate, medically known as benign prostatic hypertrophy or BPH. Half of all men in their fifties and 80 percent of men in their eighties have some symptoms of BPH. Since the prostate surrounds the urethra, these symptoms not surprisingly include dribbling after urination or a need to urinate often and especially at night.

In addition to BPH, some common prostate problems are prostatitis (an inflammation of the prostate, usually caused by bacterial infection) and prostate cancer (a common but sometimes deadly cancer that responds best to treatment when detected early).

There has been a lot of controversy recently about the use of the prostate-specific antigen (PSA) test as a screen for prostate cancer. An expert panel in the United States says not to bother while many GPs, urologists and patient advocates say "absolutely." I'm in the middle. As a stand-alone test, the PSA test is not very valuable. However, it has a role to play in conjunction with other tests.

Let's look briefly at the history of this controversial diagnostic tool. The PSA test was originally developed as a way to tell whether prostate cancer was recurring in men already treated for prostate cancer. Research has shown that in many respects the velocity and vector (rising trend past normal) of the change is more important than the one-off high reading. But since PSA levels begin to rise early in the course of prostate cancer, it was postulated that the higher a man's PSA level, the more likely it was he had prostate cancer.

With the PSA test in hand, doctors began giving the test to healthy men with no symptoms of prostate cancer. By 1991, well over a year before the start of the first large clinical trial designed to see if PSA screening actually saved lives, routine PSA screening had become widespread throughout North America. The controversy developed largely because PSA blood levels go up for reasons other than cancer—including the enlarged prostate that often accompanies age—and high readings (even one-offs) are seeing clinicians send patients for biopsies and other invasive testing.

The PSA debate rages on because we don't have a truly accurate marker to identify men who have prostate cancer that could eventually cause serious problems. Otis Brawley, chief science officer of the American Cancer Society, says, "It is very well accepted that 40 percent to 60 percent of localized prostate cancers that we cure are in men who did not need to be cured." And in fact, about 80 percent of men eighty years and older go to their graves *with* prostate cancer but not *because* of prostate cancer. The prostate typically does a good job of "walling off" cancer and keeping it from spreading to the rest of the body. Yet we continue to diagnose a large number of men without having the precise knowledge to spare those who don't actually need treatment, including drastic surgery that can result in impotence, incontinence and blood clots.

We're not without recourse at this point. A proper physical (including a good history of recent symptoms, family history and digital prostate exam) and blood cancer screening are both good diagnostic tools. Blood cancer screening includes testing for circulating tumour cells (CTCs) and for a marker known as tFFDP (tumor fibrin and fibrinogen degradation products). Both are well known by-products of cancer cells. Monitoring CTCs involves looking for cells in a blood sample that have broken free from the tumour. More studies are needed, but it may be a more reliable way to assess the status of prostate cancer than the PSA (prostate specific antigen) test alone. The fFFDP is also a simple blood test. When most cancer cells grow, they release enzymes called thrombin and plasmin that break down the neighbouring tissue to make space for the cancer cells to grow into. This type of tissue degradation is unique and specific to cancer cells and it can be measured to provide evidence to physicians about the presence of cancer. There are more than one thousand research articles supporting the association of tFFDP with cancer.

To watch a clip about prostate support, scan the QR barcode above into your smart device or enter the following link into your browser: http://bit.ly/NsgkG3

And there are in fact some ways to tweak the PSA test itself to try to get better results. It's actually possible to test two forms of PSA at once: *free* and *attached*. BPH and other non-cancer conditions tend to increase the free form, while cancer tends to produce more of the attached form. Though more research is needed, measuring free vs. attached PSA may help determine whether a prostate biopsy really is necessary. And perhaps your doctor will soon make use of all four tests we've discussed: free PSA, attached PSA, CTC and tFFDP.

Sexual Dysfunction

One group of sexual dysfunctions—sexual desire disorders, sexual arousal disorders and orgasm disorders—may occur in either men or women, with a complex range of possible causes, both psychological and physical, many still unknown. The same may be said for sexual pain disorders, which are experienced almost exclusively by women. Erectile dysfunction, of course, is exclusively a male burden.

Erectile dysfunction or ED is the inability of a man to attain or sustain an erection sufficient for sexual intercourse. It can be a persistent medical condition, although almost half of all men experience ED occasionally. Many investigators used to believe differently, but most now accept that physical factors are responsible for the majority of ED cases, with psychological factors and

To watch a clip about sexual support, scan the QR barcode above into your smart device or enter the following link into your browser: http://bit.ly/MEC4ic

drugs accounting for most of the rest. Several physical conditions may contribute to ED by impairing blood flow to the penis. These include atherosclerosis, diabetes, hypothyroidism, multiple sclerosis and chronic alcohol abuse.

Embarrassment—on the part of both physician and patient—has in the past been a deterrent to treatment, where any treatment existed. Much of that has changed now and most sufferers from sexual dysfunction will find their way to a medical professional, who will be better equipped than in the past to recommend treatment or make appropriate referrals.

TESTING HORMONES

Whether you are moving through menopause, dealing with premenstrual syndrome, looking to prevent breast cancer or trying to get pregnant, it is essential to evaluate your hormones in the most effective way possible. Men too face hormonal issues, since hormones protect and regulate the prostate, play a role in erectile function and dysfunction, and also have a crucial role in generating libido in both men and women.

Hormone issues can lead to a variety of clinical symptoms including but not limited to hot flashes, night sweats, irritability, irregular periods, sexual difficulties and brain fog. All too often however, these issues are addressed solely as hormone problems. But it's important to consider the possible involvement of nervous, endocrine and immune systems. The nervous system is the central regulator of the endocrine system, which controls hormone output and balance. The immune system can override both. Many scientists, researchers and clinicians believe that this link between the nervous and endocrine systems can lead to an increase in hormone-related symptoms if the nervous system becomes imbalanced due to stressors on the body.

Doctors often put people suffering from hormone imbalances on prescribed hormone replacement therapy and this may indeed be beneficial in managing certain symptoms. However, it does not necessarily address the possible root causes. We really need to evaluate all three of these systems to arrive at the correct diagnosis and treatment plan. That's why I've discussed immune system testing earlier and will be discussing nervous system testing later.

One of the best ways to evaluate hormone levels, whether you're a man or a woman, is to test the urine. Hormone levels naturally fluctuate over the course of a day and the measurement of hormones in urine collected over several hours provides a stable average of hormone levels that overcomes the "snapshot" limitation inherent in blood and saliva testing. Testing urine also allows us to evaluate how hormones are used through the organ cells of the body. Steroid hormones, for example, are produced primarily in the adrenal cortex, ovaries and testes, but extensively metabolized in various tissues. How they are used and broken down influences their ultimate effect and this can vary significantly person to person and day to day. Finally, the majority of hormones floating in the blood are bound to proteins that help to maintain these hormones in a non-active or "captive" form. Only the tiny, unbound fraction is useful at any given time. The concentration of hormones held in "captivity" can vary, making it impossible to predict the amount of useable hormone from a measurement of total hormone levels in the blood. Hormones measured in the urine best represent the unbound, or bioavailable, and usable form.

I said at the start of this chapter that it would be far from a comprehensive catalogue of human health issues and what follows is not a comprehensive list of hormones that can be tested via the urine. But these are some important ones that are related to both sexuality and other health aspects.

Adrenal hormone evaluation might be considered for patients with blood sugar imbalances and metabolic syndrome (elevated blood pressure, cholesterol, sugar, and fat tissue), tissue-wasting disorders or low bone density, chronic fatigue, immune dysfunction, hypo- or hypertension, allergies, menstrual irregularities or simply a history of chronic psychological or physiologic stress. Assessing adrenal hormones is also useful in people with low thyroid activity (hypothyroidism).

Corticotropin-releasing hormone (CRH) is released from the hypothalamus in the brain during stress but also in response to low cortisol indirectly, via the pituitary. CRH stimulates secretion of cortisol from the adrenal gland. High amounts of glucocorticoids also inhibit the secretion of thyroid-stimulating hormone (TSH). One of the best tests available for assessing whether cortisol levels are elevated is the measurement of "free cortisol" in a twenty-four-hour urine collection.

Adrenal stress hormones such as adrenaline render your cells and tissues less sensitive to the effects of your thyroid hormone. This can cause weight gain and fatigue. In light of these effects, addressing adrenal imbalances before administering thyroid hormone makes sense and may help improve tolerance of medication in those people who end up requiring it.

Thyroid hormone is one of the primary drivers of basal metabolic rate. The most sensitive indicator of whether the thyroid gland is working effectively is the amount of TSH (thyroid stimulating hormone) that is required to be produced by the pituitary gland. If the thyroid is flagging, most commonly because of an autoimmune attack, TSH rises above normal in order to raise the thyroid hormone level. There has been some controversy recently regarding the "normal range" of TSH.

To watch a clip about thyroid support, scan the QR barcode above into your smart device or enter the following link into your browser: http://bit.ly/LC5o2v

Androgens are known as the "male" hormones but found in both men and women, with much higher levels in males. Their evaluation should be considered for those experiencing decreased libido or sense of well-being, bone loss, signs and symptoms of "andropause" in men (i.e., loss of muscle mass, increased fat tissue especially in the waist, decreased sex drive and motivation). Excessive androgen in women may result in excess hair growth especially on the arms, legs, chin and upper lip, spotted hair loss on the crown of the head, and chin line acne. A history of polycystic ovarian syndrome (PCOS) may be an underlying cause worthy of further investigation.

Estrogen and progesterone (or more accurately its metabolite called *pregnanediol*) levels can be tested to evaluate ovulatory function in pre-menopausal women with menstrual irregularities and/or infertility. Knowing these levels can also help assess menopausal symptoms in peri- or postmenopausal women. Estrogen metabolites help assess the risk of breast or prostate cancer, osteoporosis (in postmenopausal women not using HRT) and autoimmune conditions such as lupus and rheumatoid arthritis. If you are taking natural supplements such as indole-3-carbinol (I3C), diindolylmethane (DIM) or sulforophane, then testing for these markers is helpful in monitoring whether or not they are working for you at the dose (and type) you are currently using.

I've talked about the complex interrelationship of hormones and that's why I often recommend—at least initially—that patients have a comprehensive urinary test that consists of all of these hormones. You can employ smaller panels or individual tests for follow-up testing to monitor your response to treatments or to check levels of previously abnormal results.

4. PUMPING IRON

OUR HEART AND THE BLOOD IT MOVES

You'd really have to have been dozing most of your days to have missed the enormous emphasis public health education places on cardiac health. And the more emphasis, the better, because so many of us are in denial about our risk factors for heart disease. Each year, about 250,000 potential years of life are lost in Canada due to cardiovascular diseases, including stroke, heart attacks and other chronic heart-related conditions. A whopping nine out of ten people are jeopardizing the quality and length of their lives. In this section, we're obviously going to explore heart health but we're going to look a little deeper too.

The heart is so important because it's the pump that drives blood through the body and it's our blood that is the medium of life. Blood carries the vital nutrients to every cell and carries away the toxic wastes. But the critical reaction that produces energy—and energy is life—requires more than fuel; it needs oxygen to burn the fuel and this task too is entrusted to our blood. So when a little later in the section we come to talk more about testing, you'll see we're interested in not just the heart but the vital supplies that are carried in our blood.

Cardiovascular Health

In an ideal world, time would be spent screening patients for heart disease. Sadly, a recent poll conducted by the Canadian Heart and Stroke Foundation found that about 50 percent of Canadians hadn't even been asked by their doctor about their diet, family history of heart disease or stroke, weight, level of physical activity, or even whether they smoked. And yet there is an irrefutable connection between genes, diet, exercise and heart disease.

To begin taking charge of your heart health, there are three crucial measurements I want you to track and optimize routinely with your family doctor. If you can become more aware of them and strive to adjust them to optimal levels, you'll live longer and keep a healthier heart for that longer life.

Blood pressure. About 1 in 6 people have high blood pressure or hypertension and 1 out of every 3 aren't aware they have this serious medical condition. You want to have less than 140 over 90 at all times (except while exercising when a modest rise in blood pressure is normal).

Waist size and fat percentage. If your waist (which is not where your belt sits but is above your hips but below your ribs) is more than 35 inches as a woman or 40 inches as a man, your risk of dying prematurely is nearly double. Get accurately checked for your body fat percentage using something called impedance analysis. Don't over-rely on the famous body mass index (BMI) since it doesn't distinguish between muscle, fat and water.

Updated blood work. Get checked regularly for blood cholesterol levels, fasting sugar levels and High Sensitive C-reactive protein (HS-CRP).

Together, blood pressure, waist size, fat percent and CPR measures give you a good basic risk assessment of heart health.

If all of these are even slightly high along with a slightly elevated blood pressure, you may not only be at risk for heart disease but also at elevated risk for diabetes, whether it runs in your family or not.

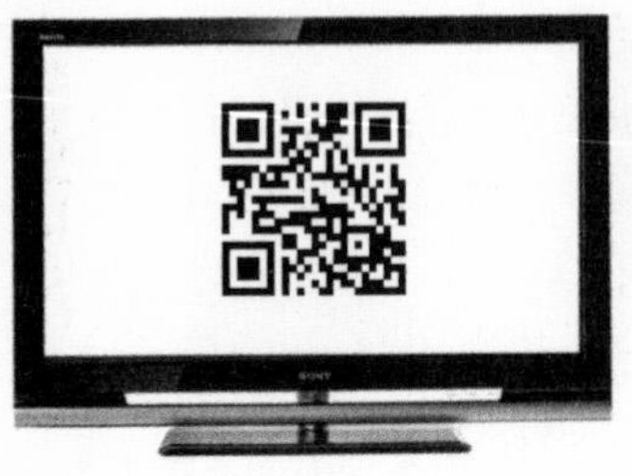

To watch a clip about heart health and cardiovascular support, scan the QR barcode above into your smart device or enter the following link into your browser: http://bit.ly/NN1UyX

Anemia and Red Blood Cells

If you're experiencing fatigue, lethargy, weakness, poor concentration or frequent colds, you may have a condition called anemia. Anemia is a general term for a category of blood conditions that affect the red blood cells or the oxygen-carrying hemoglobin they contain.

In people with anemia, there is either a reduction in the number of red blood cells in circulation or a decrease in the amount or quality of hemoglobin—the oxygen-carrying molecule that has an iron centre. There are many causes of anemia, including iron deficiency, severe blood loss, genetic disorders and serious diseases. Anyone with unexplained anemia should have the cause determined by a qualified doctor. Some athletes appear to have anemia when their blood is tested, but this may be a normal adaptation to the stress of exercise, which likely doesn't need treatment. You should *not* supplement with iron, however, unless a blood test has revealed a true deficiency. Often a simple blood test called a complete blood count or CBC will determine the underlying issue. But be sure to also ask your doctor to include B12 levels as well as ferritin, which tells you about the amount of *stored* iron in your body.

To watch a clip about red blood cell support, scan the QR barcode above into your smart device or enter the following link into your browser: http://bit.ly/LG5eqU

Blood Sugar

Hypoglycemia, also termed "low blood sugar," occurs when the level of sugar carried by the blood drops too low to provide energy sufficient for the body's activities. In adults or children older than ten years, hypoglycemia is uncommon except as a side effect of diabetes treatment, but it can result from other medications or diseases, hormone or enzyme deficiencies, or tumours.

To watch a clip about blood sugar support, scan the QR barcode above into your smart device or enter the following link into your browser: http://bit.ly/QdMF4Y

Normally, the body makes insulin when it is needed. Right after meals, the body produces enough insulin to process the blood sugar from that meal, moving it out of the blood and into the cells. Between meals, the level of insulin drops before it can drive blood sugar levels too low. If there is not enough insulin to allow glucose to enter the cells, too much glucose remains in the blood. This can cause symptoms of diabetes, including fatigue, frequent urination, thirst and a risk of ketoacidosis (a dangerous condition with warning signs that include rapid deep breathing and sweet-smelling breath, or breath that smells like nail-polish remover). Hypoglycemia can occur if the individual has more insulin than normal, has eaten too little food, or has been unusually active. Indeed, exercise helps insulin work more efficiently. These days, testing for insulin levels is important for many people, not just the diabetic.

Blood Pressure

Blood pressure is the force of blood pushing against the walls of arteries (blood vessels). Each time the heart beats, it pumps blood through blood vessels, supplying the body's muscles, organs and tissues with the oxygen and nutrients that they need to function.

To watch a clip about high blood pressure support, scan the QR barcode above into your smart device or enter the following link into your browser: http://bit.ly/P4LW2G

When your doctor takes your blood pressure or perhaps when you do it yourself at the local pharmacy, there are two numbers of importance: the systolic and diastolic numbers (also referred to as the top and bottom numbers). The top number, systolic blood pressure, measures the maximum pressure exerted as the heart pumps blood outward, while the lower number indicates diastolic pressure, a measurement taken between beats, when the heart is at rest. The World Health Organization suggests that ideal blood pressure sits at 115/75 mmHg.

Approximately two-thirds of people over the age of sixty-five have high blood pressure. Of all people with high blood pressure, 61.4 percent are under current treatment, 35.1 percent have it under control, and 64.9 percent do not have it controlled. Hypertension, or a blood pressure that exceeds normal for any prolonged period of time—roughly anything more than 130 over 90—must always be evaluated by a health-care professional. Extremely high blood pressure or rapidly worsening hypertension almost always requires treatment with conventional medicine. People with mild to moderate high blood pressure should work with a professional before attempting to use natural health products.

Cholesterol and Health

Has any natural body substance suffered worse PR than cholesterol? This soft, waxy, fat-like substance is found within the bloodstream and cells of the body and its synthesis is a naturally occurring process that is essential to produce membranes for all cells, including those of the brain, nerves, muscles, skin, liver, intestines and heart. Cholesterol is also converted into steroid hormones, such as the male and female sex hormones and the adrenal hormones. In the liver, cholesterol is the precursor to bile acids that aid in the digestion of food, especially fats, and is a key component in the body's manufacture of vitamin D.

Yet, alas, according to current estimates, high levels of blood cholesterol affect about 20 percent of adults over the age of twenty in North America. Too much cholesterol in the blood is a major risk for heart disease, which may lead to a heart attack, during which the heart cannot pump enough blood to the body, and premature death. High cholesterol levels are also a risk factor for stroke, which occurs when not enough blood and oxygen get to the brain. Surprisingly, the highest prevalence occurs in women between the ages of sixty-five and seventy-four. The World Health Organization (WHO) reports that high cholesterol contributes to 56 percent of cases of coronary heart disease worldwide and causes about 4.4 million deaths each year.

High cholesterol can cause the formation and accumulation of plaque deposits in the arteries. Plaque is composed of cholesterol, other fatty substances, fibrous tissue and calcium—normal substances in the blood that become deposited on the artery walls when there is inflammation or injury to the artery wall. Studies show that people whose LDL cholesterol is made up of predominantly small, dense particles have a risk of coronary heart disease that is three times greater than the baseline. And now there are tests to measure LDL particle size.

To watch a clip about cholesterol support, scan the QR barcode above into your smart device or enter the following link into your browser: http://bit.ly/OUu3zQ

If your cholesterol levels are too high, you will want to work towards achieving optimal levels as soon as possible. First, to determine what those levels are, speak to your family doctor about running some fasting blood work, which could include CBC, total cholesterol, HDL and LDL, LDL particle size, triglycerides, HS-CRP, homocysteine, ApoA1 and B and ionized calcium. Be aware that the majority of the cholesterol in the body is manufactured by the liver and is NOT related to dietary consumption.

TESTING YOUR BLOOD: BEYOND CHOLESTEROL

Most of us know by now that maintaining a healthy diet guarantees that our blood will carry all the necessary vitamins and minerals our bodies need to function optimally.

To watch a clip about vitamin support, scan the QR barcode above into your smart device or enter the following link into your browser: http://bit.ly/MXwQb7

Right? Hmmm . . . maybe not. Good scientific studies have shown that it is virtually impossible to achieve all our nutritional needs from diet alone. If you're reading this book, you probably understand already that true nutrition—not just satisfying hunger—is important to human health. In fact, nearly 80 percent of North Americans take vitamins and supplements in order to feel better and prevent disease.

Of course the foods we eat have an impact on our bodies. Eating junk food for a month, for example, can increase a person's cholesterol levels significantly. The foods we do *not* consume also have an impact on our bodies, and even eating too much of a good thing has an impact on our bodies. Try eating ten pounds of broccoli in one day and see if you feel healthy.

But for all this common sense, we still can't be sure how much *each one of us* requires of each known nutrient—unless, of course, we test ourselves. Some of the diseases and conditions affected by nutrition are ADD/ADHD, fatigue, heart disease, periodontal disease, autoimmune disease, intestinal symptoms (bloating, diarrhea, gas), diabetes, joint inflammation and pain, lung disease, kidney disease, depression, macular degeneration, cataracts, infertility, liver disease, Alzheimer's, Parkinson's, poor wound healing, eczema, cancer and allergies—and that's just to name a few. Whether you have any or a combination of these ailments—or you're lucky enough to have none at all—it's important to understand which supplements are right for your body, your lifestyle and your circumstances. Your goal is to ensure that your unique needs are met without wasting money on stuff that could be unnecessary or even harmful.

To watch a clip about multivitamins, scan the QR barcode above into your smart device or enter the following link into your browser: http://bit.ly/NRLcvu

Let's do a quick survey of the blood nutrients that are most important, the ones whose levels you need most to be concerned about, and the ones you most need to test for. They are: antioxidants, B vitamins, essential and toxic minerals, and amino acids.

Antioxidants

Antioxidants are the famous protective molecules that reduce the damage to our cells caused by the highly reactive but naturally occurring molecules called "free radicals." This damage is sometimes referred to as oxidative stress. Antioxidants are essential for this defensive role and they make an important contribution to the healthy function of our neurological, hormone and immune systems. In fact, I wrote an entire book on their importance—*The Antioxidant Prescription: How to Use the Power of Antioxidants to Prevent Disease and Stay Healthy for Life*. In it I describe how oxidative stress is linked to premature aging, heart disease, neurological diseases and chronic fatigue syndrome. If your levels of

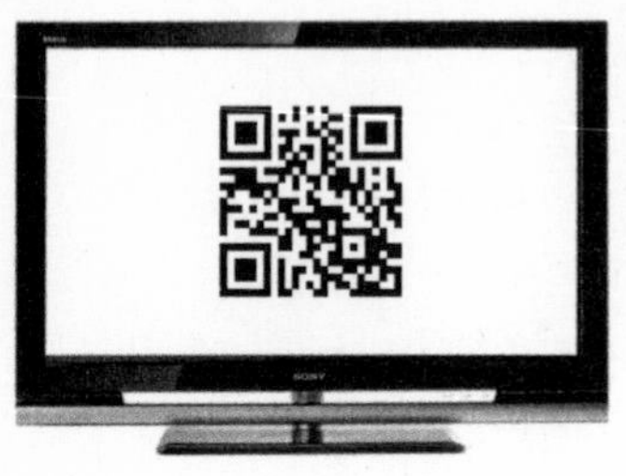

To watch a clip about antioxidant support, scan the QR barcode above into your smart device or enter the following link into your browser: http://bit.ly/OXs15J

antioxidants are low, you're less protected from these harmful compounds. There are now tests available that assess the necessary equilibrium between oxidative stress and antioxidant protection. Among the most important antioxidants whose levels we need to assess are CoQ10, alpha lipoic acid (ALA), and vitamins A, C and E.

B Vitamins

B vitamins are essential for energy, metabolism, weight loss and nervous system support, among other things. It is important to test all of these levels when assessing general health. B1 is a required co-factor for enzymes involved in energy production from food and for the synthesis of ATP, the body's currency of energy. B2 is a key component of enzymes involved in antioxidant function, energy production, detoxification and vitamin activation. B3 is used to form NAD and NADP, which play a role in energy production from food, fatty acid and cholesterol synthesis, cell signalling and DNA repair. B6 (or P5P) is a co-factor for enzymes involved in carbohydrate metabolism, the manufacturing and synthesis of neurotransmitters (our brain chemistry), red blood cells and their heme (necessary for oxygen delivery) and your DNA. B7, or biotin, is a cofactor for enzymes involved in the manufacture of fatty acids, cellular energy and DNA activity. B9 (a.k.a. folic acid) plays a key role in coenzymes involved in DNA synthesis, methylation (essential for heart and nervous system health), amino acid metabolism and red blood cell production. B12 plays important roles in energy production from fats and proteins, methylation, synthesis of hemoglobin and RBCs, and the maintenance of nerve cells, DNA and RNA.

Amino Acids

Amino acids are integral to healthy body chemistry. They serve as the body's basic building blocks and are responsible for the production of bone and muscle. Balance is critical for proper nerve function, metabolism, detoxification and digestion. When certain amino acids are too high or low, the result can be fatigue, increased risk for cardiovascular problems, and impaired mood and cognitive function. Once identified, imbalances can be corrected, helping to prevent many chronic illnesses before they can cause severe and lasting damage.

Essential and Toxic Minerals

Minerals in our body serve two functions: they are the body's building blocks and they are regulators of our body's processes. Many of these minerals are derived from the diet, and sometimes minerals are added to the diet as supplements. Some minerals, for example, magnesium, copper and manganese, are necessary and beneficial. If proper amounts are not obtained, problems such as joint pain, weight gain, depressed libido, depression or anxiety can occur. On the other hand, exposure to mercury, lead, arsenic and certain other metals can be harmful, causing fatigue, emotional disturbances and even kidney failure. Testing for both essential and toxic minerals can provide extremely valuable information about your health.

Your Heart's in Your Genes

It's time again to visit our now-familiar friends the SNPs (single nucleotide polymorphisms), those variations in our genes that affect our individual destinies. This time we're concerned with the genes that balance blood pressure, regulate cholesterol, metabolize nutrients, mitigate inflammation and deal with oxidative stress.

Again, through genetic testing, we can gain unprecedented insight into what we need to do to prevent mutated genes from acting up prematurely. If you knew which of your genes had mutated and needed more of your attention, you could alter your diet, get better control of your stress, exercise more or supplement appropriately—and put years on your life.

Here are some key heart-related genomic tests: *apolipoprotein E* (ApoE) plays a key role in cholesterol regulation by helping to remove dietary cholesterol from the bloodstream. Scientists know that mutations in the gene that is responsible for ApoE can contribute to Alzheimer's and premature cardiovascular disease. There are a few variants called alleles: ApoE2, ApoE3 and ApoE4.

The ApoE2 allele is quite common; it shows up in approximately 15 percent of the population and is associated with lower LDL cholesterol (the bad stuff) and higher HDL (the good stuff), but unfortunately comes with a predisposition to higher triglycerides (as found in metabolic syndrome and diabetes). The E2 type also has a lower risk of atherosclerosis, myocardial infarction, stroke and osteoporosis, and higher antioxidant activity than other types. So, should you discover that your genes express the E2 type of Apo, the cholesterol-lowering effects of a low-saturated-fat and a low-cholesterol diet will be less effective for you. For you, minimizing high-sugar foods, which produce the largest triglyceride response, may be the best dietary approach. Dietary fibre, fish oils and exercise generally improve the lipid profile in this genotype also. Omega-3 fish oils reduce triglycerides most effectively in E2-type people and they also generally respond the most favourably to the statins—the most popular cholesterol-lowering medication. The E2 population also responds to a more natural supplement routine using inositol hexaniacinate, red rice yeast and policosanol. Consider the significance of this as an example of supplementation based on genetic testing. You discover you're an E2 type and realize that by supplementing with an antioxidant such as inositol you could significantly reduce your chances of developing heart disease. This method of treatment is nothing short of revolutionary.

APO E3 is the most common allele while APO E4 carries the highest risk of developing Alzheimer's and cardiovascular disease especially if one carries two copies of E4. Fortunately the latter group also responds well to conventional medications to lower bad cholesterol.

E-selectin interacts with specialized white blood cells through the lining of blood vessels. This interaction is a critical and early event in the development of atherosclerosis—plaque build-up in arteries. If you have mutations in the gene that controls E-selectin, it can drastically affect cholesterol metabolism and you may experience early onset of complications related to blood coagulation. Should testing suggest that you have an elevated genetic susceptibility, I would recommend an increase in your intake of omega-3 fatty acids (which are inversely related to E-selectin levels), a strict avoidance of trans fats, and quitting smoking *now* (smoking significantly increases E-selectin expression in blood vessels). You might also consider natural estrogen support, which would reduce E-selectin levels post-menopausally, and ensure that you're an ideal weight, because E-selectin tends to be high in obese individuals.

MTHFR is a key enzyme in folic acid metabolism and helps to create a required nutrient that manages homocysteine—a molecule that has damaging effects to the cardiovascular system. Mutations of the gene that controls MTHFR may impact neurotransmitter metabolism, reduce your coenzyme Q10 levels and even alter synthesis of your DNA.

Individuals with this genetic risk for altered folate production have increased risk of autism, depression, neural tube defects, cardiovascular disease, diabetic retinopathy, osteoporosis and some cancers. Should you find that this SNP is part of your genetic inheritance, you'd want to ensure adequate intake of folate-rich green vegetables. You would also seriously consider supplementation with folic acid (or folinic acid or 5-methyltetrahydrofolate), vitamins B2, B3, B6 (pyridoxal 5-phosphate), B12 (or methylcobalamin) and betaine (trimethylglycine) as part of your daily routine. In other words, you'd take a high dose B-complex and regularly check your levels. Remember, your genes don't change but the blood levels of the enzymes they express can and do change.

Guanine nucleotide-binding protein. G-proteins work to regulate cell-to-cell communication in the body. A mutation in this gene may give rise to increased risk of essential hypertension, atherosclerosis, myocardial infarction and enlargement of the left ventricle in the heart. There is also increased risk of obesity, insulin resistance and depression. For people who discover they have this variance, there is usually a favourable blood pressure response to clonidine, thiazide diuretics, calcium channel blockers and sodium restriction. When it comes to natural medicine, there is also typically a favourable response to taraxacum (dandelion), which acts as a natural diuretic. It's not all bad news, though. People with a G-protein mutation also exhibit a greater immune response to hepatitis B vaccination and conventional treatments for hepatitis C and HIV, and a favourable response to antidepressant treatment, regardless of class, *and* a greater erectile response to Viagra.

AGTR1 mediates the effects of a naturally occurring chemical called angiotensin II (AGT II), which relates to contraction of blood vessels, inflammation and oxidative stress. When mutated, there is a significant risk of hypertension, coronary artery disease and kidney disease. There is, however, typically a more favourable response to calcium channel blockers in this group and to the nutrients that minimize the effects of AGT II, which include fish oils, borage seed oil, magnesium, potassium, L-arginine and L-taurine.

Plasminogen activation inhibitor-1 (PAI-1) is one of the factors in charge of coagulation of blood and is found in blood platelets as well as in the walls of blood vessels. Its job is to increase clotting when necessary. When this mechanism isn't working well due to genetic mutation, then higher PAI-1 levels occur and there is an increased risk of thrombosis (blood clots). There is also a possible increased risk of gum disease (periodontitis), asthma and allergic disease, and polycystic ovarian syndrome (PCOS) in females. There can also be an increased risk of obesity, especially in post-menopausal women. When genetic mutations on genes that control this enzyme are found, it becomes important to evaluate insulin resistance. Weight reduction and regular exercise become key, since these regimens will naturally reduce PAI-1. A plan to minimize stressors and reduce one's intake of saturated fat and alcohol is imperative. If warranted, the "ACE inhibitors" (angiotensin-converting-enzyme inhibitors), which are pharmaceutical drugs used primarily for the treatment of high blood pressure, are particularly effective in people who express this genotype and have high blood pressure. Hormone therapy and supplementation with dehydroepiandrosterone (DHEA) reduces PAI-1, decreasing clots post-menopausally. The naturally derived fermented soy supplement called "nattokinase" dissolves fibrin and manages elevated PAI-1.

5. THE LIFE OF THE MIND: SOME THOUGHTS

The nervous system is the vital link between our internal and external worlds. The sense organs receive external stimuli and relay this information to the brain, which processes it and passes instructions to our organs, tissues and cells, allowing them to manage and adapt to changes in our environment.

To watch a clip about brain and mood support, scan the QR barcode above into your smart device or enter the following link into your browser: http://bit.ly/LJrgOn

Profound neurological diseases such as Parkinson's, and profound mental disorders such as schizophrenia are not well defined within the scope of natural medicine—and indeed no system of medicine has conquered them. But there are many aspects of everyday mental health that we will be considering, and the heartening news is not only that therapies have advanced in these areas, but also that tests to measure and assess these conditions are now available to many more of us.

TESTING NEUROTRANSMITTERS

You may be currently experiencing, or previously may have had, a confusing set of symptoms that your doctor wasn't able to figure out. Perhaps you became convinced that the symptoms were "all in your head." The thing is, you may have been more right than you knew.

Neurotransmitters are recognized as the primary biochemical messengers of the central and peripheral nervous systems; they are in charge of our thoughts and emotions. Many health concerns are the result of improper neurotransmitter signalling. Think about your own health. What's been bothering you? Headaches, anxiety, poor sleep or fatigue? Or, maybe you're experiencing intestinal complaints or have recurring illnesses. These and many other symptoms may be the result of imbalances in one or more neurotransmitters.

Knowing the source of imbalance is crucial in order to select the right intervention or supplementation. There is now a body of scientific literature that demonstrates that the measurement of neurotransmitter chemicals in the urine has clinical value because these neurotransmitters are biomarkers of various neurological, immunological and endocrinological conditions. These studies have demonstrated that measures of urinary neurotransmitters are reflective of circulating levels. In other words, urinary measures are not recognized as a *direct* measure of central activity, but definite correspondences are now thought to exist.

If you're extremely fatigued, it may be that your brain's glutamate, norepinephrine and epinephrine are out of whack. People who experience excessive anxiety often have imbalanced taurine. Those suffering depression and general low mood typically have depressed serotonin levels. Attention difficulties are often associated with dopamine imbalance. If you have cravings that lead to improper eating habits and other weight management difficulties, serotonin, glutamate and dopamine may be involved. Intestinal complaints may be associated with serotonin; poor cognitive function may be linked to PEA and dopamine. Headaches may involve serotonin and histamine. Immunity malfunctions may point to imbalances in serotonin, glycine, glutamate, histamine and norepinephrine. If your issue is poor sleep, the neurotransmitters serotonin, GABA, glutamate, PEA, norepinephrine and epinephrine may all be involved.

Let's look at each of these a little more closely.

Stress, Anxiety and Adrenal Fatigue

To start with, let's define how we're going to use these words. For our purposes, "stresses" are external factors that place demands on our system. They are challenges, and as such we may perceive them as positive (such as the stress of competition in sport), but more frequently they affect us in a negative manner. "Anxiety" is the unpleasant experience of worry, dread or fear that is sometimes our response to stress.

There is no greater impact on the brain, the nervous system and our chemical neurotransmitters than *intense emotional or severe physical stress*. The way in which you perceive stress (a very subjective thing) and the way you *manage* stress throughout your life can have a substantial impact on your health and well-being. Modern living can sometimes create stresses that the body can no longer adapt to. People who have trouble coping with stress often have systemic health issues such as inflammatory or immune problems as well as neurotransmitter imbalances. For such people, more effective coping with stress is of critical importance.

The Natural Standard organization defines *anxiety* as "an unpleasant complex combination of emotions often accompanied by physical sensations such as heart palpitations (irregular heart beat), nausea, angina (chest pain), shortness of breath, tension headache, and nervousness." I would add fatigue, insomnia, stomach problems, sweating, racing heart, rapid breathing, irritability and even depression.

We commonly focus anxiety on events that *may* happen. Of course, some anxiety about stressful future events is normal, but human reactions to stress vary enormously. Some people experience little anxiety until they're at the receiving end of a major catastrophic event. For others, everyday anxiety interferes with their ability to function. We say that these people suffer from an "anxiety disorder" and they often have symptoms that go beyond a simple response to stressful situations. Such anxiety disorders are characterized by constant worry or panic, avoidance of certain situations, and nightmares or flashbacks to a traumatic event. Sufferers may experience a racing heart, panic, trouble sleeping or obsessive thoughts, and may go so far as to avoid social situations. This level of anxiety can be disabling or even dangerous.

It's important for those who suffer from an anxiety disorder to seek expert medical care, and the caregiver's first step before considering an appropriate treatment plan is to determine the cause of the symptoms. For instance, just as with depression and ADHD/ADD, scientific study has determined that chronic inflammation is often found in individuals with anxiety issues. Inflammation affects mood by altering brain chemistry and hormones. Infections, allergies or hypersensitivities should be investigated along with neurotransmitters.

To watch a clip about brain chemistry, scan the QR barcode above into your smart device or enter the following link into your browser: http://bit.ly/QgqH1d

The third item I mention in the heading above is *adrenal fatigue*, which can be the result of remaining stressed out for too long. The term describes a cluster of symptoms—fatigue, trouble getting up in the morning, a dependence on caffeine, trouble sleeping or insomnia, weight gain, depression, cravings and poor immune function—that may be related to suboptimal adrenal gland function. Laboratory testing can look at hormones produced by the adrenal gland as well as other markers related to adrenal function.

If adrenal fatigue is suspected, laboratory evaluation is often limited to the hormones produced by the adrenal gland (cortisol and DHEA). But adrenal fatigue can only be properly evaluated if neurological and regulatory neurotransmitters affecting the adrenal gland are also assessed.

To watch a clip about stress and anxiety support, scan the QR barcode above into your smart device or enter the following link into your browser: http://bit.ly/NHdMkw

If, apart from the stark emotion of fear, you experience any of anxiety's other symptoms—difficulty coping, extreme fatigue, regular feelings of being overwhelmed, high blood pressure, irritable bowel syndrome, gastric ulcers or anger problems such as road rage—then laboratory analysis of your neurotransmitter levels may actually suggest a targeted amino acid therapy customized to your test results as well as your anxiety disorder symptoms.

Paying Attention—Or Not

Attention deficit hyperactivity disorder (ADHD) is characterized by attention difficulties and hyperactivity, while attention deficit disorder (ADD) is characterized by attention difficulties and inattentiveness. Both ADD and ADHD are common among children, who may have behavioural issues and poor grades in school. Adults too can exhibit ADHD/ADD symptoms. They may be forgetful and have difficulty meeting responsibilities and remaining organized.

It's startling to learn that chronic inflammation or infection is commonly found in individuals with attention and hyperactivity issues. Chronic inflammation affects moods by altering brain and hormone chemistry and the root causes of inflammation (infections, allergies or hypersensitivities) should be investigated as part of the health-care practitioner's standard evaluation. Food sensitivities, for example, are a common cause of attention disorders and hyperactivity in children.

There are other symptom patterns that appear related to ADHD/ADD. Switching tasks frequently, difficulty focusing on one task, general focus issues, impatience, excess energy, inability to sit still, trouble following instructions and impulsive behaviour—all suggest that an evaluation of neurotransmitters may be useful in determining the cause of these issues. Testing for imbalances in neurotransmitter levels can help to develop a treatment plan to address both the symptoms and the underlying imbalances. In many cases symptoms such as these may be accompanied by a high level of excitatory neurotransmitters. A natural approach to these imbalances is calming support both through lifestyle interventions and supplementation with amino acids.

As with ADHD/ADD, root causes such as inflammation caused by infections, allergies or hypersensitivities are prime suspects.

Depression: The Dangerous Emptiness

If you suffer from fatigue, inability to concentrate, difficulty remembering details or making decisions, strong feelings of guilt, worthlessness, and/or helplessness, feelings of hopelessness and/or pessimism, major changes in sleep patterns, irritability, restlessness, loss of interest in activities or hobbies, changes in appetite, persistent aches or pains, headaches or digestive problems, persistent sad, anxious or "empty" feelings, then you may be suffering from depression.

Depression has both physical (biochemical) and emotional causes and can occur with highly variable severity ranging from mild sadness/loss of interest, to suicidal thoughts/actions. If you feel suicidal, you need to seek professional help *immediately*. Do not wait. Depression can be a dangerous sickness.

Whatever its causes, depression always has an underlying biochemical aspect and it's very common for people with depression to follow antidepressant therapies recommended by their doctor. Assessment of neurotransmitters involved in depression can be helpful in selecting the best class of medication or supplementation, tracking the medication's effects and determining its success. Commonly prescribed medications for depression work by altering brain neurotransmitter signalling. A widely used class of drug is known as selective serotonin re-uptake inhibitors (SSRIs), whose common brand names include Celexa, Prozac, Paxil and Zoloft. These work by selectively increasing available serotonin so as to have a mood-elevating effect.

Testing neurotransmitter levels can provide valuable information about the status of the nervous system and its interaction with other systems in the body. Once the biochemical abnormalities contributing to the depression are identified, your caregiver can undertake a personalized treatment approach. New studies have led scientists to believe that chronic inflammation is commonly found in depressed individuals, just as with many of the disorders we've just discussed. Chronic inflammation affects mood by altering brain chemicals and hormones. Again, the root causes of inflammation (infections, allergies or hypersensitivities) should be investigated as part of your health-care practitioner's standard depression evaluation.

Insomnia: When the Ravelled Sleeve of Care Won't Knit

If you have trouble falling asleep, staying asleep, or if you always wake feeling unrefreshed, you may be suffering from some form of insomnia, a common medical complaint characterized by the inability to get a sufficient amount of sleep at night. Insomnia may be due either to difficulty falling asleep or to trouble staying asleep for an appropriate amount of time. People with insomnia may also have fatigue or anxiety during the day due to lack of quality sleep during the night.

Those with sleep difficulties may be taking a variety of prescription medications to assist with sleep. Most of these medications work by altering brain neurotransmitter levels. Again, testing neurotransmitter levels can be very beneficial in selecting and monitoring treatment.

Test Yourself for Neurotransmitter Levels

Again, just as with blood nutrient and enzyme levels, or hormone and mineral levels, there are non-invasive urine tests that can tell you with real accuracy what your levels are for many of the neurotransmitters we've discussed in this section. At the end of the chapter, I'll provide some contacts for testing of this sort.

6. A PAIN IN THE LIFE: THE SIGNAL WE CAN'T IGNORE

I'm including a section on pain not only because pain is central to many of the questions I am most often asked, but also because it allows me to discuss inflammation, one of the most important aspects of human health.

We can define pain as an unpleasant sensory experience associated with damage to body tissues, including organs, bones and muscles, or an unpleasant *emotional* experience related to psychological trauma. The physical damage irrefutably gives rise to inflammation but scientists are beginning to learn that psychological trauma also induces inflammation. Pain, the most common reason individuals seek medical care, is often classified as either acute (short-term) or chronic (long-term). Approximately 30 to 40 million North Americans experience pain that does not respond to over-the-counter analgesics such as acetaminophen, aspirin and ibuprofen. And some researchers have estimated that as many as 35 percent of North Americans experience chronic pain of some sort. According to the National Institutes of Health, the annual cost of chronic pain in the United States, including health-care expenses, lost income and lost productivity, is estimated to be about $100 billion. But pain is not a disease: it's a symptom. It's commonly described as the body's crucial signal to us—we need pain to keep us safe.

The four most common areas of pain are lower back pain, severe headache or migraine pain, neck pain and facial ache or pain. Back pain is the leading cause of disability in those under forty-five years old.

To watch a clip about pain support, scan the QR barcode above into your smart device or enter the following link into your browser: http://bit.ly/PMxgmm

I guess I don't need to tell you to consult with a health-care practitioner if you suffer from persistent pain of unknown origin. Pain is one of those things that almost everyone is inclined to look into. The real issue is what course you'll follow if your pain is not readily resolved. Let's survey a few common sources of chronic and acute pain. Then we'll look at the testing that can assess the underlying causes.

Arthritis

Although we commonly associate arthritis with aging, younger people can be affected, too. What characterizes almost all arthritis is the pain it inflicts on its victims. Arthritis literally means joint inflammation or swelling. Arthritis affects the joints, the tissues surrounding the affected joints and other connective tissues. The most common forms include rheumatoid arthritis and osteoarthritis

Osteoarthritis, also known as degenerative joint disease, occurs when the cartilage in the joints starts to break down. It occurs most often in individuals older than forty-five, but it may develop at any age.

To watch a clip about arthritis support, scan the QR barcode above into your smart device or enter the following link into your browser: http://bit.ly/PDJxts

Rheumatoid arthritis is an autoimmune disorder that occurs when the body's immune system, which normally fights against disease and infection, attacks itself. Unlike osteoarthritis, which only affects the bones and cartilage, rheumatoid arthritis may also cause swelling in other areas of the body.

Women are two to three times more likely to develop either form of arthritis than men. However, rheumatoid arthritis may also develop in young children and older adults.

Fibromyalgia: The Mystery Pain

The main symptom of fibromyalgia is chronic, widespread, musculoskeletal pain—general pain and stiffness throughout the body—for which no obvious cause (such as tissue inflammation or damage) can be identified. The cause of fibromyalgia is unclear but current theory is that it may be the result of a central nervous system malfunction, resulting in amplification of pain transmission and detection. Common additional symptoms can include: fatigue, sleep disturbances, headaches and facial pain, as well as depression, anxiety and difficulty concentrating.

To watch a clip about fibromyalgia support, scan the QR barcode above into your smart device or enter the following link into your browser: http://bit.ly/MEpa3D

Scientists at the National Institutes of Health (NIH) estimate that fibromyalgia affects five million Americans eighteen years of age or older. The vast majority of fibromyalgia cases are women from their mid-thirties to late fifties. However, men and children can also have the disorder. An estimate of the prevalence of fibromyalgia is as high as 3 to 5 percent of the population in North America.

Toothache

I suppose toothache just about defines what we mean by pain in an everyday context. It enjoys a reputation for being just about as bad as pain can be without being life-threatening. Most instances of toothache are caused by a dental cavity, a cracked tooth, an exposed tooth root or gum disease. The severity of a toothache can range from chronic and mild to sharp and excruciating and the pain may be aggravated by chewing or by cold or heat.

If you experience tooth pain, a thorough oral examination by your dentist is required. It may include dental X-rays that can help

To watch a clip about toothache support, scan the QR barcode above into your smart device or enter the following link into your browser: http://bit.ly/MBvelf

OR

To watch a clip about ear care support, scan the QR barcode above into your smart device or enter the following link into your browser: http://bit.ly/QfSr65

determine whether the toothache is coming from a tooth or jaw problem and identify the cause. If you need an X-ray, you may wish to take alpha lipoic acid, which can act as a protective agent against the minor amount of X-ray radiation that you receive during the investigation.

I should mention that sometimes a toothache may be caused by a problem not originating from a tooth or the jaw. Pain around the teeth and the jaws can be symptoms of diseases of the heart (such as angina or heart attack), ears (such as inner or external ear infections) or the sinuses. Infections and diseases of the ears and sinuses can also cause pain around the teeth and jaws. An evaluation by both your dentist and your doctor may be necessary to diagnose the seemingly simple "toothache."

INFLAMMATION TESTING: SPOTTING THE SMOKING GUN

Inflammation is a general term to describe the accumulation of fluid, plasma proteins and white blood cells in an area of the body where there is injury, infection or some sort of tissue damage. Inflammation may be acute, as for instance in the type that influenza can suddenly cause in the lungs, or chronic, as in the case of an autoimmune disease such as arthritis. No matter what type of pain or discomfort you may be in, and no matter what type of disease you may have or be predisposed to genetically, inflammation is playing a role—and if it isn't already, it will.

Testing with hs-CRP and ESR

We have a number of reliable tests for detecting inflammation and drawing out information about the underlying cause.

If your doctor suspects that you have an acute condition causing inflammation—a serious bacterial or fungal infection or an inflammatory disorder such as arthritis, or an autoimmune disorder or inflammatory bowel disease—he or she can order up a high-sensitivity C-reactive protein test. This simple blood work can identify the presence of inflammation and monitor response to treatment for an inflammatory disorder. Sometimes it's used simply to screen patients for any inflammation that may be brewing—a sort of cellular fishing expedition.

An erythrocyte sedimentation rate (ESR) may be ordered along with the CRP when a condition or disease is suspected of causing inflammation somewhere in the body. Because an ESR can detect evidence of numerous inflammatory conditions, it may be ordered when arthritis is suspected of causing inflammation and pain in the joints, or when digestive symptoms suggest inflammatory bowel disease. ESR is an easy, inexpensive, nonspecific test that has been used for many years to help detect conditions associated with acute and chronic inflammation, including infections, cancers and autoimmune diseases. Like CRP, ESR is said to be "non-specific" because it can be affected by conditions other than inflammation, and even if inflammation is actually present, elevated levels do not tell us exactly where the inflammation is in the body or what is causing it. For this reason, both CRP and ESR are typically used in conjunction with other tests.

Testing Cytokines

Inflammation is not all bad. It rids the system of dead or infected or damaged tissue and cells and prevents the spread of infection. Inflammation is part of the call to arms that gets as many immune cells to the affected area as possible and resolves the problem quickly and efficiently. And we've already encountered the messengers who sound the alarm that starts the whole process: the cytokines.

Our inflammatory responses result in detectable changes in the cytokine levels in our biological fluids such as serum and plasma. These changes, which vary according to the disease or threat involved, make cytokines valuable for testing. Elevated or diminished cytokine levels are associated with many clinical conditions and diseases including central nervous system disorders, autoimmune disorders, infections, allergies, asthma, fibromyalgia and diabetes. Imbalances may also be harbingers of cancer, heart disease, obesity, depression, severe pain and all sorts of classic inflammatory disorders.

In the section on invasion and response, we looked at cytokines that stimulate the immune system to eliminate bacteria and help signal for the elimination of virus-infected cells. Other cytokines can promote harmful conditions such as allergy and asthma and certain autoimmune disorders. But taken as a whole, cytokines work to ensure tolerance, balance and regulation of immune response.

Cytokine testing can identify the presence of both an activated immune response and a suppressed immune response. It can guide targeted therapeutic regimens designed to reduce inflammation and its secondary effects, or to address a poorly functioning immune system. Natural medicine is often noted for its advocacy of potent remedies that can boost immune function, but boosting an already hyperactive immune system can make matters worse. It's generally more important to *balance* the immune system and cytokine testing is a tool that can help point us in the right direction.

Stimulated Cytokines

White blood cells that produce elevated cytokines are strong indicators of inflammation. Yet paradoxically, people with chronic illness, who are undoubtedly suffering from the effects of inflammation, usually have only mildly elevated serum cytokine levels. In this situation another measuring tool, stimulated cellular cytokine analysis, can make a real contribution.

Stimulated cytokine analysis is performed by subjecting the patient's white blood cells to agents such as a plant-derived product called phytohemagglutinin (PHA), which stimulates T-cells, or lipopolysaccharides (LPS), which use components derived from a bacteria to switch on the parts of the immune system—the macrophages and B cells—that munch up bacteria. By stimulating the white blood cells of the immune system using PHA or LPS, and then comparing the stimulated responses of these white blood cells to a baseline using specialized laboratory instrumentation, we're able to learn more about the ability of a person's immune cells to respond appropriately. And we can determine the presence of inflammation—and the type of inflammation. From there, we can decide how to deal with it.

7. A MATTER OF YEARS: THE RAVAGES OF TIME

Aging is not in itself a disease. The three most observable signs to aging—*deterioration* (wrinkles, lines and larger pores), *descent* (drooping and sagging, courtesy of the laws of gravity, which makes us look tired and worn) and *deflation* (the hollowing-out loss of contour)—might be best thought of as age-related effects superimposed on the actual aging process but not actually identical to it.

A great deal of research has been devoted to aging and longevity and intriguing pieces of the puzzle are showing up everywhere. Studies of centenarians have found anomalously high levels of vitamins A and E and the enzymes glutathione reductase and catalase. Long lives seem to be linked to heredity, a healthy diet, lots of exercise, more education and an extroverted personality.

But is it really possible to arrest aging? Can we even hope to slow it? Can we, in other words, *anti*-age?

All the explorers are back in port and the news is, no fountain of youth was found. What we've caught glimpses of, though, is the possibility of medicines and practices that might add another twenty or thirty healthy years to our lives. Recent scientific studies have been changing much of our knowledge about what makes us grow old too fast and what makes us stay young longer. A really comprehensive discussion of aging is way beyond the scope of this book, so before we look at some of the latest thinking on the subject, let's just mention a few afflictions that we commonly associate with getting older. Many of these overlap with issues we've discussed under the topic of hormones, blood nutrition and brain chemistry. How could it be otherwise? The entire human organism is woven together, so every part seems to interact with every other part.

My Poor Old Bones

Contrary to popular belief, bone is living tissue, not inert material. Bone in fact is one of the most active tissues in the body, constantly being broken down and rebuilt in a process called remodelling. Like any other living tissue, it needs nourishment to stay strong and healthy as we age.

Bone cells use proteins and other building blocks to produce a substance known as collagen, whose fibres develop quickly to form an organic mesh that calcium, magnesium, phosphorus and numerous other minerals attach to. Without the ideal levels of minerals and nutritional building blocks, your body cannot create the strong, finished, hardened material we recognize as healthy bone. The opposite—weak, porous bones—is a condition we call osteoporosis.

Bone loss accelerates suddenly in menopausal women because of reduced estrogen levels, causing an increase in the resorption of existing bone, but resorption is only half of the story. Age-related bone loss is caused by a decrease in the formation of new bone tissue (due to many factors including nutrition and the cumulative loss of the piezoelectric effect through lack of exercise). Bones need mild impact to stay healthy. Ample evidence from space exploration shows that astronauts lose considerable amounts of bone when their bodies are in a zero gravity environment for extended periods of time. Existing drugs for osteoporosis and supplements such as calcium and vitamin D supplements work to increase the mineralization of bone but they do not help the body to build new bone tissue. Within weeks of starting use of antiresorptive drugs like Fosamax, the body's formation of new bone actually *decreases*. The resulting bone is less prone to fracture, but is not the same as youthful, healthy bone.

As with so many other health issues, we have reason to believe that nutrition plays a vital role in bone health. Are we getting that nutrition? Blood calcium and phosphorus tests are available through your physician, but these are for the most part inaccurate as assessments of the current health of your bones. Bone density testing is important to determine bone health, but is not particularly effective at determining osteopenia—the beginning of the bone loss process—and by the time they can detect osteoporosis, it's hard to remedy. Technology has to improve substantially in the area of bone density analysis before it can be

To watch a clip about building stronger bones and bone support, scan the QR barcode above into your smart device or enter the following link into your browser: http://bit.ly/P3UaYZ

considered something to implement in a preventive manner. However, a simple blood test for vitamin D levels early on is an excellent way to ensure you have enough of that vital nutrient to provide bone-building support. The appropriate vitamin D test is called 25-hydroxy-vitamin D or 25OHD and the optimal or target blood level is between125–250 nmol/litre.

The Energizers

Energy equates with life and we equate low energy with illness and age. No energy at all is death. There are plenty of well-known synthetic ways to obtain energy in the short run, but all of these shortcuts call us to account sooner or later. The challenge is to achieve energy naturally.

Mitochondria: The Energy Factories

Deep within every cell of our body, mitochondria are the tiny power plants that generate the energy we need to live. Without the required amount of mitochondria we fade, tire, droop and die. Many advances have been made in our understanding of the role mitochondria play in health, disease and aging and, in fact, their activity—their energy output—can be tested. The most sensitive and specific test for mitochondrial dysfunction is an organic acid analysis of urine. Organic acid testing can detect dysfunction of mitochondrial energy production as well as the presence of functional nutrient deficiencies and toxins that are adversely affecting detoxification pathways.

The Adrenals: Ever Ready

Our bodies have evolved to run on energy regulated by our adrenal glands, our bodies' rechargeable batteries. As we've seen, stress is not only North America's number one silent killer through its effects on the heart, but it zaps our energy by draining our adrenals. When you learn how to recharge your adrenals you reduce your chances of heart disease and find more energy.

And stress and worry start in the brain. When stress levels become more than a person can handle, three brain chemicals—serotonin, noradrenalin and dopamine—are used up faster than they can be made. We've met some of these neurotransmitters before and it's no surprise that the subjective effect of their loss is a significant drop in our mental, emotional and physical energy.

When we're frightened or stressed our adrenal glands release adrenaline and another hormone called cortisol into our bloodstream. Our heart beats faster, blood flow is shunted away from our skin and intestines and towards our muscles. Perspiration appears on our palms and forehead. We're ready for "fight or flight." A cousin of adrenaline named noradrenalin is the "happy hormone," the messenger that sets our energy levels. Proper functioning of it in the brain is essential for that energized feeling, but when too much adrenaline circulates for too long, it wastes noradrenalin; its levels fall and we feel exhausted, tired, droopy and without energy. We just don't feel like doing anything. We just want to sit. Sitting causes the metabolic cog wheels to slow down and eventually grind to a halt. When that happens, the signal to the body is to more quickly get ready for its own demise.

To watch a clip about energy and stamina support, scan the QR barcode above into your smart device or enter the following link into your browser: http://bit.ly/P4AfJh

To watch a clip about hormone support, scan the QR barcode above into your smart device or enter the following link into your browser: http://bit.ly/LIMbfJ

Moans and Hormones

And, of course, hormones are back and that's no surprise either. Hormones are produced by our pituitary, hypothalamus, adrenals, thyroid and gonads. They control everything from our reproductive functions to our mood, our sleep, our appearance—indeed, almost every aspect of daily life. It has become common to blame various problems on our hormones and in fact there's a little truth in this. These streams of hormonal output must remain in balance with one another in order to optimally regulate our physiological, psychological and emotional reactions. If you drag yourself out of bed in the morning, if you have uncontrollable sugar cravings or chronic headaches, if you lack energy or get stressed out by the slightest thing, the underlying cause may be a hormonal imbalance. This sort of imbalance tremendously increases the risk of conditions associated with aging: cancer, diabetes, osteoporosis and heart disease. If our hormones *are* in balance, however, we have the potential to reach one of life's most attractive goals: to age gracefully and remain youthful to the end.

To watch a clip about inflammation support, scan the QR barcode above into your smart device or enter the following link into your browser: http://bit.ly/MAY1wl

Inflammation: The Universal Affliction

Inflammation too is back by unpopular demand. We know it normally as the visibly raised, red, hot, swollen and painful area around an injury—not itself a disease but part of the body's natural response to harmful stimuli such as infection and irritants. Its role is to protect the affected tissue and initiate healing. Sadly, the story doesn't stop there. I'm introducing the subject of inflammation in this section on aging because its unfortunate negative effects can accumulate in time and be far more pervasive than once thought. No matter what your ailment—from headaches to heart disease and joint pain to Alzheimer's disease—scientists have discovered that inflammation is often at the root. At the cellular level, chronic inflammation has the effect of turning on bad genes and predisposing you to everything from diabetes to cancer.

The Retreat of Muscle.
The Advance of Fat.

Metabolic Syndrome

Metabolism is the sum of the chemical reactions that take place within our bodies' cells to sustain our lives. *Metabolic rate* is the rate at which our metabolism expends energy, both at rest and when active, and thus the rate at which the body burns its substance (usually fat). This is a vast subject, but our concern here is with so-called *metabolic syndrome,* which we ran across when we were talking about hormones and about the blood. We can define metabolic syndrome as an unhealthy ratio of body muscle to body fat. I'm broaching this subject again, this time under the broad heading of aging, but metabolic syndrome is most certainly not confined to the elderly—we can see this plainly just by walking down the street. Yet our metabolism *does* slow with age and many people who were slim in their younger years struggle with excess weight as they age.

As is now widely recognized, North America is in a state of health emergency: an obesity epidemic in which more than 60 percent of us are overweight and 25 percent are considered obese. Even more alarming is the fact that approximately 20 percent or more of us don't even realize that we need to lose

To watch a clip about body composition, scan the QR barcode above into your smart device or enter the following link into your browser: http://bit.ly/QtHCwf

excess body fat. And you aren't safe just because you appear to be of normal weight. Despite looking relatively trim, many people have altered or unhealthy body composition, that is, they carry too much fat tissue relative to lean tissue such as muscle. The consequences of unhealthy body composition are many and they are very similar to obesity: heart disease, hypertension, back pain, high cholesterol, stroke, sleep apnea and metabolic syndrome, to name a few. Metabolic syndrome affects about 46 percent of the North American population and is characterized by high blood pressure, high cholesterol, high blood insulin and glucose levels and, as a rule, a waist circumference greater than 40 inches for men and 35 inches for women. These factors significantly increase the risk of type 2 diabetes, heart disease and stroke and are all easily measured by a competent practitioner. Recent studies are also finding a significant association between metabolic syndrome and Alzheimer's disease. And since estrogen can be produced by fat tissue, our hormonal balance too can be affected by unhealthy body composition

Amino Acid Deficiency

Alanine, arginine, glutamine, glycine, tryptophan and tyrosine are all amino acids, and as such they're among the building blocks from which the body creates the proteins necessary for life. There are twenty standard amino acids in the genetic code. Combinations of these amino acids produce every essential protein needed for the human body's healthy balance. Most bodily processes cannot occur without amino acids because those processes require the proper protein to function.

There is a good amount of scientific opinion that holds that the body may in some cases fail to manufacture certain amino acids. To know whether you would benefit from taking amino acids, consider asking your health-care provider to run a laboratory test that quantifies levels of circulating amino acids and their metabolites, and evaluates essential and non-essential amino acid nutrient status in the blood.

Some Acidic Observations

Most of us are aware that plants require the soil in which they grow to have a specific balance of alkalinity and acidity if they are to thrive. We may not think of such balances as required by our own bodies, but in fact human homeostasis, as it is called, is essential to life. The osmotic pressure of bodily fluids, the sugar levels in the blood, the iron levels, the temperature levels and many other factors must be kept in careful balance by the body's mechanisms. One of these, like the pH of soil, is the acid-base balance in our bodies. If this balance is lost, proteins are denatured and digested, enzymes can no longer function, and death may result.

The term "pH" doesn't stand for "potential of health," but it might as well. It actually stands for the "potential of hydrogen." I'll spare you the chemistry, but we should talk about why pH is important to our health. The potential of hydrogen (pH) is based on a scale. There is a tenfold difference between each number going from 1 (most acidic) to 14 (most alkaline). In general, the body tissues and systems work at a *neutral* pH of 7 (or very close to it) and the blood is only slightly alkaline. Any extended disturbance in the acid-alkaline balance, by only the tiniest amount, will cause major problems.

For years it has been speculated that an alkaline diet is one that promotes a lean, healthy body. Recently there have been studies supporting this hypothesis. The first, published in the

To watch a clip about pH support, scan the QR barcode above into your smart device or enter the following link into your browser: http://bit.ly/MjFvWQ

British Journal of Nutrition (2008), showed that among more than 1,100 young women, there was a strong association between a more acidic diet and a greater risk of being overweight. In this study, both body mass index (BMI) and waist circumference were positively associated with acid-forming foods. Additional research shows that higher BMI, in turn, may promote a more acidic environment in the human body. A diet consistently high in acid-forming foods is an obstacle to maintaining lean muscle mass, especially after age sixty, and a loss of muscle mass appears to be an adaptive response to a consistently acidic diet. Older persons are most vulnerable to the effects because the elimination of acidic hydrogen ions through the urine is less efficient through the aging process. In a study of almost four hundred older adults, a more alkaline urine was associated with a greater lean body mass percentage. This supports a preliminary study where short-term alkalinity (accomplished by potassium bicarbonate supplementation for the purposes of the study) had a favourable effect on lean body mass in just eighteen days.

The Acid Diet

Until recently, the importance of dietary influences on pH has been grossly underestimated. Our diet is fairly heavily weighted towards the acidic and the health implications of a consistently acidic diet now appear to be broad ranging. In the *British Journal of Nutrition* study mentioned above, it was demonstrated that among more than 1,100 young women, there was a strong association between a more acidic diet and a greater risk of being overweight. New evidence suggests that being more systemically alkaline may help prevent cancer. An acidic diet appears to promote oxidative stress (the kind caused by free radical molecules) and inflammation, draws calcium and magnesium from the bones, promotes the production of stress hormones and encourages fat storage. No wonder it's suspected of influencing many chronic conditions, from cardiovascular disease to osteoporosis, from obesity to the visible signs of aging.

To watch a clip about testing your pH, scan the QR barcode above into your smart device or enter the following link into your browser: http://bit.ly/MESd7b

Acidosis. If our cells are constantly exposed to an acidic environment, we are in danger of developing a condition known as acidosis, in which our arterial pH falls below 7.35. Studies have shown that an acidic, anaerobic (oxygen-deprived) body environment encourages the breeding of fungus, mould, bacteria and viruses. It is a lot of hard work for our body to neutralize and detoxify these acids before they can act as poisons in and around the cells, ultimately changing the environment of each cell. If the body can't keep up, our inner biological terrain shifts from a healthy oxygenated, alkaline environment to an unhealthy acidic one and begins to set up defence mechanisms to keep the damaging acid from entering our vital organs. Here are some symptoms that you may be surprised to learn can stem directly from the root cause of acidosis:

Overweight. It is known that acid is stored in fat cells. As a defence mechanism, the body may protect itself from potentially serious damage by creating fat cells to store the acids and keep these wastes at a safe distance from the vital organs. Many people have found that a return to a healthy alkaline biological terrain helps them to drop excess fat.

Joint pain and arthritis. All substances left by the metabolizing process are acidic and toxic; therefore these have to be neutralized by alkalizing elements such as calcium ions, sodium ions and lithium ions, of which calcium is the most important. Calcium ions are positively charged ions that are constantly looking to combine with acids to form calcium carbonate. Calcium carbonate is harmless and will be moved out of the body if our body fluid pH is alkaline. Otherwise, the calcium carbonate is deposited around skeletal joints, leading to numerous health problems such as pain or arthritis.

Osteoporosis. Many people think they can eliminate osteoporosis by increasing their consumption of milk and dairy products. But in fact the incidence of osteoporosis is low in countries where the consumption of dairy products is low. Osteoporosis is actually an acidosis problem. As the body becomes more acidic, our body tries to remain healthy to protect us against heart attacks, illness, strokes or even cancer. To do so, it takes calcium from the teeth, bones and tissues, making them weak and brittle.

Underweight. Yeast and fungus produced in an acidic environment can feed on our nutrients and thus reduce the absorption of everything we eat by as much as 50 percent. Without adequate protein the body can't produce the enzymes, hormones and other chemical components necessary for cell energy and organ activity. We can become very thin as a result and this is no healthier than being overweight. As alkalizing and oxygenating takes place, the body naturally begins to seek its own ideal weight.

Low energy and chronic fatigue. An overly acidic environment causes our biological terrain's oxygen level to drop, leaving us tired and fatigued. This will allow parasites, fungi, bacteria, mould and viral infections to flourish and gain a hold throughout the body.

Heart attack. If bacteria and/or fungi and/or viruses attach themselves to the inner walls of arteries under the influence of an acidic body environment, this can attract white blood cells, causing proteins and cells to clot forming a plaque in the artery that narrows it and restricts the flow of blood, nutrients and oxygen to the tissues. Should that happen to a coronary artery, a heart attack can occur.

Allergies. The toxins produced within an acidic, oxygen-deprived environment coupled with the absorption of undigested proteins can be a major cause of allergy conditions. When the digestive system is weakened, a wide range of allergic reactions can occur, e.g., food allergies, and the overall susceptibility to allergens is increased.

Acne. There are many different forms of acne, and not a few are linked to an unhealthy diet, especially diets that are highly acidic.

Frequent colds, bronchitis, infections, headaches. Only when our pH level is fairly balanced can oxygen bind efficiently to the hemoglobin protein of our red blood cells in the lungs. If the pH is too acidic, microbes in our respiratory systems can grow far more easily, causing bronchitis, pneumonia and sinusitis, and invading our cell system. The result can be chronic cough, bronchial spasms (asthma), colds, infections and headaches.

Testing Our pH

Established testing called the potential renal acid load (PRAL) analysis determines how particular *foods* may have an acidic or alkaline effect *inside* the body. It is now well documented that the current Western diet is heavy in acid-forming foods that score a high positive PRAL. Scientists have estimated that the ancestral human diet had a urinary PRAL of (-)39 per day, far more alkaline than a typical present-day urinary PRAL of (+)23. Overall, the daily acid production in the body of modern North Americans is at least three times higher than in pre-agricultural humans, contributing to a lot of the chronic diseases we suffer from.

There is no single way to test our body's pH. Any general deviation, however small, from the blood's proper pH balance will result in death if not corrected quickly and hospital emergency rooms can conduct arterial blood gas analysis that can tease out the main causes of such acute acidosis. Blood pH generally will not otherwise fluctuate enough to test. However, the body's pH can be tested via urine or saliva, and a skilled clinician will always take into account the time of day and your hydration level before considering the value of your urinary or salivary pH. The general rule of thumb is you want to be higher than a pH of 6 on urine or higher than 7 on saliva.

CLOCKING OUR SPEED OF AGING

Real Age

One of the most striking findings of recent research is that most of us aren't direct reflections of the number of candles on our last birthday cake. Prominent American physician and author Dr. Michael Roizen talks about what he calls the "real age" factor. He means that most of us have a chronological age and a biological age. He offers an online test at www.RealAge.com that suggests that some of us are a lot older while some are a lot younger than the number that appears on our driver's licence. The variables are things like your personal medical history, your family history, your stress levels, whether you take your vitamins and get enough nutrients, your attitude toward life, and of course the quality of your sex life. (Wouldn't want to omit that.) The test takes minutes. I'm a real fan of Real Age—but not *only* because while I'm approaching forty the test results tell me that my body is still looking forward to its thirtieth birthday party!

Good for you, you might say. But why are any of us aging at all?

Oxidation

Aging studies are only beginning to scratch the surface and science hasn't yet settled confidently on a comprehensive theory of what causes our bodies to age. However, one of the most interesting theories points to free radical damage as an underlying mechanism of aging. Science may someday eliminate today's leading killers of older people, but different maladies will take their place and most of them are likely to be linked to free radicals, those dangerous little oxygen molecules we've already encountered and that star in my last book, *The Antioxidant Prescription*. Free radicals are largely the result of the body's normal metabolism but they unfortunately wreak havoc on our cells. Free radical damage begins early and eventually exceeds the body's self-repair capabilities, gradually impairing the functioning of cells, tissues, organs and organ systems, increasing vulnerability to disease and giving rise to the familiar manifestations of aging: loss of muscle and bone mass, a decline in reaction time, compromised hearing and vision, greying of hair, reduced elasticity of the skin.

The interaction of free radicals with your DNA produces genetic destruction. The body deals with this destruction by invoking DNA repair enzymes to remove damaged genetic material. This destruction can be tested for. Free radical damage of guanosine (simply put: a piece of DNA) produces 8-hydroxy-2'-deoxyguanosine (8OHdG). The concentration of 8OHdG in urine has been shown to be an accurate measure of the rate of DNA damage (more specifically known as polynucleotide oxidative damage). Elevated 8OHdG is a sign that antioxidant nutrient intake may need to be increased. Toxins and lifestyle stress factors as well as excessive physical activity may contribute to increased oxidative challenge.

Telomeres: The Life Fuses

As though the attacks of the free radicals weren't harrowing enough, in the last four years scientists have discovered that our very genes carry a mechanism that may make aging inevitable. Dr. Elizabeth Blackburn won the Nobel Prize in 2009 for her discovery of telomeres, which are little disposable buffers at the ends of our chromosomes. When the chromosomes replicate, as they must do if their DNA message is to survive a good long lifetime, the telomeres are gradually worn away to protect the information at the ends of the genetic message. When a cell's telomeres have finally worn away entirely, the cell stops dividing and enters a senescent stage and eventually dies. So telomere length is theoretically correlated directly to biological age and any comparisons to the fuse of a bomb are appropriate since the shorter our telomeres are, the sooner we hit our expiry date. That's biological aging, folks, and it doesn't sound that encouraging, does it? However, the truth can set us free—or at least give us a few more years of freedom. It's actually possible to test the average telomere length on lymphocyte blood cells from a sample of the population in the same age range. The higher the telomere score, the "younger" your cells.

This is such a key measure, I'm recommending that you should have telomere length testing done once per year to evaluate the rate of aging. In Chapter Four, we'll focus on telomeres in greater detail, to learn what we can do to slow the burning of this "life fuse."

TEST YOURSELF: BLOOD NUTRIENTS, TOXINS, ENZYMES, HORMONES AND BRAIN CHEMISTRY

It was only a matter of time before modern laboratory testing became accessible to ordinary people without their having to access the often cumbersome medical system—a system that doesn't always provide biological testing for individuals looking to know their personal nutrient, hormone and toxin levels, as a measure of how healthy they are. I am pleased and proud to be part of that process.

The alternative health and supplement world is vast and within it there are some dubious claims that need to be examined with great care. One of my main goals in communicating with the public is to be a trustworthy guide and authority on everything that's out there. In a multi-billion-dollar supplement product industry, it's time consumers knew whether a natural health product has really been assessed for safety and effectiveness before deciding whether to spend their hard-earned dollars on it. To rely on product testimonials or even a "proven research" claim—which in actuality may be a study done on all of nine people—is inadvisable at best. The only real way to know what you need more or less of is to get tested using the latest technology.

My own company, Wylde About Health, Inc. has recently joined forces with two world-class CLIA-certified laboratories to be able to provide at-home urine and saliva testing that reveal your personal supplement needs.

I am *not* in the business of developing a personal supplement line—nor will I ever be. I've turned away many offers to use my brand likeness on the front of a supplement line. My company, Wylde About Health, Inc., has, however, made much of the testing I discuss above available so that anyone can understand with real accuracy what their current health status is related to their nutrient status. The MyStatus™ test kits give you, the consumer, the power to learn your personal levels of vitamins, minerals, hormones, antioxidants, toxins, brain neurotransmitters and much more. The results are for educational and research purposes only. The MyStatus™ test kit results generate custom supplement plans that detail only those things *you* require in order to help prevent the onset of disease and better manage your individual health concerns. There's no need to go to your family doctor to obtain these results, because this non-invasive test simply requires a urine or saliva sample or, in some cases, a drop of blood from your finger. The MyStatus ™ kit comes with biological collection containers and simple step-by-step instructions. For babies and newborns, pediatric diaper collection bags are supplied.

You can learn more details about MyStatus ™ testing at www.wyldeabouthealth.com/mystatus. If on the other hand you're considering getting tested through your family doctor or natural health-care practitioner, here are some other laboratories that I have great confidence in, with some descriptions provided by the companies themselves.

GENOVA DIAGNOSTICS LABORATORIES (www.gdx.net)
Genova Diagnostics is a fully accredited medical laboratory, certified in the areas of clinical chemistry, bacteriology, mycology, parasitology, virology, microbiology, non-syphilis serology, general immunology, hematology, toxicology and molecular genetics by six separate health agencies, including the Centers for Medicare & Medicaid Services which oversee clinical labs in the United States under the federal Clinical Laboratory Improvement Amendment (CLIA). Including myself, Genova serves more than 8,000 other primary and specialty physicians and health-care providers. Established in 1986, the lab offers more than 125 specialized diagnostic assessments, covering a wide range of physiological areas including digestive, immunology, metabolic function and endocrinology.

NEUROSCIENCE, INC. (www.neurorelief.com)
NeuroScience, Inc., offers assessments for neurotransmitters and neuromodulators, hormones and neuroimmune markers through the laboratory services of Pharmasan Labs, Inc. Established in

1999, NeuroScience is a research- and education-driven company committed to improving human health. In conjunction with Pharmasan Laboratories, NeuroScience, Inc. provides laboratory assessments and clinical tools in the fields of neurology, endocrinology and immunology. Dr. Gottfried Kellermann, Chairman, CEO and founder of NeuroScience, Inc., has been offering neurotransmitter assessments since 1999 and has worked with healthcare practitioners to assess nearly half a million individuals.

METAMETRIX LABORATORY (www.metametrix.com)
Metametrix provides clinical laboratory services in the area of nutrients, toxicants, hormonal balance, biotransformation and detoxification, gastrointestinal function and the microbiome. Their service, as with the above labs, helps to custom tailor nutritional therapies, detoxification programs and other lifestyle changes for the prevention, mitigation and treatment of complex chronic disease. Metametrix is recognized internationally as a pioneer and leader in the development of nutritional, metabolic and toxicant testing and they have introduced several firsts to the industry, including quantitative organic acid analysis to identify nutrient and other metabolic imbalances; quantitative fatty acid analysis; fingerstick technology as a non-invasive option, and DNA identification of gut microbes.

ROCKY MOUNTAIN ANALYTICAL LABORATORY (www.rmalab.com/)
Rocky Mountain is the only accredited laboratory in Canada providing wellness testing services specifically for practitioners of complementary and alternative medicine. They are the first accredited Canadian laboratory to offer saliva hormone testing commercially and do the saliva testing in Canada. As a renowned saliva hormone testing facility, they also provide testing for allergies, adrenal, thyroid and insulin resistance conditions.

AXYS ANALYTICAL SERVICES LTD. (www.axysanalytical.com)
AXYS conducts ultra-trace analysis of persistent organic pollutants and emerging organic contaminants. The company has focused exclusively on emerging contaminants for thirty years and has experience in environmental, human, biota and food matrices that they claim "ensures legally defensible analysis" for clients who may need regulatory analysis of legacy pollutants such as dioxins and PCBs, specialized analysis of emerging contaminants such as PFCs and PBDEs, or method development for compounds of new concern like pharmaceuticals and personal care products and hormones and sterols.

DOCTORS' DATA, INC. (www.doctorsdata.com/home.asp)
Doctors' Data, Inc. (DDI) is a licensed CLIA laboratory with appropriate state certifications. The company participates in numerous quality assurance/proficiency testing programs including those of the College of American Pathology, New York State DOH and Le Centre de Toxicologie du Québec. The company has thirty years' experience and provides specialty testing to healthcare practitioners, especially toxic elemental testing of multiple human tissues. The laboratory offers an array of functional testing. Their tests are utilized in the assessment, detection, prevention and treatment of heavy metal burden, nutritional deficiencies, gastrointestinal function, hepatic detoxification, metabolic abnormalities and diseases of environmental origin.

NAVIGENICS (www.navigenics.com)
Founded in 2006 by David Agus, M.D., an oncologist, and Dietrich Stephan, Ph.D., a human geneticist, the company's clinically guided genetic testing services are based on research initially made possible by the Human Genome Project, a thirteen-year federal and international collaboration to identify every single

human gene. Navigenics' website states that they "believe that genetic testing and analysis will become the foundation and standard of care that will make personalized medicine a reality."

COUNSYL (www.counsyl.com)
Counsyl's mission is to scale up the Jewish community's successful campaign of universal carrier screening for Tay-Sachs, which vanquished the disease by 2003. To do this, Counsyl seeks to make preventive carrier testing universally accessible and to use their resources to find cures and treatments for families suffering from genetic disease. The organization was founded by social entrepreneurs and philanthropists with the belief that "every child deserves a chance in life."

TESTING WITHOUT TESTS

After our brief survey of areas of health concern and the many new and exciting opportunities to throw light into areas of health that were formerly dark, I'd like to wrap up this chapter by looking at some time-honoured and uncomplicated "tests" that have long provided insight.

A "biomarker" is an observable change that indicates an underlying state of health or disease: the presence of antibodies, for example, that suggest a present or recent infection, or sugar in the urine that signals the possibility of diabetes. In some cases, a biomarker may point to a disease before the disease itself appears. Familiar examples are blood lipid levels—cholesterol and triglycerides—used by doctors to assess the risk of future heart disease. Our bodies, like our cars, have warning lights. If, when your oil warning light flashed, your first impulse was to open the hood and disconnect the annoying thing and then chug on down the highway, the result would be a disaster—for the car. Biomarkers can be these flashing signs of compromised body systems. We must know how to read these signs.

To watch a clip about biomarkers and how your body talks, scan the QR barcode above into your smart device or enter the following link into your browser: http://bit.ly/PCjG8H

To watch a clip about skin, hair, and nail support, scan the QR barcode above into your smart device or enter the following link into your browser: http://bit.ly/NNETvN

But our bodies offer an array of biomarkers that require no lab tests at all; they're observable physical signs of stress that may signal a risk of potential illnesses requiring treatment. Doctors have been observing them for centuries so let's end the chapter by looking at a few.

Hair, skin and nails play a particularly telltale role because they are affected over time by your state of health.

Look at your hair. If it has lost its shine, it may be an indication that you are low on essential fatty acids. You should be supplementing your diet with essential fatty acids such as fish oil. If you are greying prematurely, it may suggest you are low on para amino benzoic acid. If your hair is falling out, check your iron levels and thyroid but you may also want to consider supplemental B vitamin.

Look at your nails. Some people's fingernails show lots of white spots. If you don't have reason to believe that the white marks came by way of injury, this could be an indicator that your body needs more calcium or zinc. If you have vertical ridges (called "Beau's lines") in your nails, your digestive enzymes—especially hydrochloric acid—may be low or you're taking too high a dose of antacid medicine. If your nails break easily, consider the amino acids glutathione and NAC, and try the mineral silica.

Look at your hands. If you're prone to warts, taking a combination of vitamin A and beta-carotene may help. If you have dry hands, use lots of hand cream, wear gloves in the winter and increase your fish intake for the EFA content—especially deep-water fish such as fresh or canned wild Alaskan salmon, sardines, farmed rainbow trout, albacore tuna, Atlantic mackerel, black cod or farmed arctic char. These fish are among the healthiest you can eat; they are relatively clean and free of chemicals and heavy metals.

Alas, not all biomarkers are as easily observed as these. I wish they were. That's why we've devoted this chapter to the search for hidden signs. We may not be as well as we think, though we're getting better and better at correcting this shortsightedness.

Now, in the chapter that follows, let's see what we can do with what we've learned about ourselves.

CHAPTER 3

—

GETTING HEALTHY

SOME REMEDIES CONSIDERED

Not a day goes by that I don't field a health question from somebody desperate to try an alternative or complementary remedy that might help them back to a state of health. I get pummelled by questions during a busy day in clinic; I get pulled over on the street; I do live television where I answer viewer call-ins; I get hundreds of e-mails (I welcome anyone to submit a question to me and my expert team at www.wyldeonhealth.com/ask); and I often receive private calls from a friend of a friend's cousin who wants an effective solution for their arthritis or diminished energy or a complement to their chemotherapy treatment.

I'm honoured that so many come to me with their health

questions and concerns, knowing that I keep up on all the newest and most advanced testing, products and services in the natural health industry. I was recently asked to be part of the inaugural medical advisory board for *The Dr. Oz Show*—and I didn't hesitate for a moment to accept the invitation as one of the alternative medicine specialists. As always, I am wholly committed to being a trusted and informed voice for all those who seek my advice. In the previous chapter, we looked at testing in seven areas of common concern. In this chapter I want to provide you with concise information about a selection of natural health products that address those same concerns. It's all based on what *you* want to learn more about. I'll especially focus on products I've had experience with in my clinical practice and feel qualified to express an opinion about. These are always supported by scientific databases and peer-reviewed medical journals, articles and research.

The natural health industry is riddled with junk science, fuelling my desire and priority to "debunk the junk." My primary motive is to empower consumers to make appropriate educated choices in the realm of natural and complementary alternative choices that are often found over the counter at your local pharmacy or health food store. When you hear countless anecdotes about human growth hormone supposedly slowing down the aging process; raspberry ketones that miraculously drop fat pounds; noni juice, acai berry and mangosteen(all of which are touted as having incredible healing effects and cancer prevention properties); coconut water that replenishes our cells better than anything on the planet—well, what are you to believe? Indeed, very few products that the supplement industry promotes are "A-level." While I could never cover every worthy supplement or remedy with good science to back it, I've put my emphasis here on remedies of merit.

If you're reading this book, you're an inquiring person with a real interest in your health. It's my hope that the relatively small number of natural health solutions I describe and evaluate here will inspire you to look into the subject further, exploit the great resource of the Internet and ask questions of your own health care provider. In fact, on my own website, www.wyldeabouthealth.com, I have a free database with over half a million pages of searchable information on the topic of natural medicine. Please accept my invitation to plunge into this resource.

For many of the remedies that appear in this chapter, I've provided a rather simplistic rating based on five factors: claim, scientific validation, cost, ease of compliance and cautions with use. I of course relied on my own clinical experience, but I've also consulted a number of accepted authorities. I especially considered whether the product in question was recognized by the Natural Health Products Directorate (NHPD) in Canada, which has the highest standards in the world, and also considered whether the U.S. Food and Drug Administration (FDA) had approved it or not. I based each rating on a scale of 20, where the higher the number, the better. In the case of cost, 20 is the most cost-effective. In the case of cautions, 20-rated remedies merit the highest confidence in their safety. I chose 20 because it allows a maximum score of 100 for the five factors combined and somehow I find it easier to compare percentage scores. Must be something to do with school.

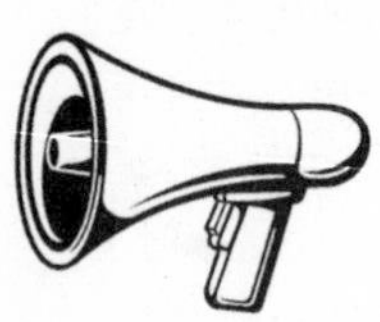

The Claim

A true claim of moderate efficacy obviously trumps a dubious claim of astounding results—and both can be difficult to quantify. I offer my own and others' experience and have given considerable weight to the Natural Standard organization (www.naturalstandard.com). A 20 represents my solid support for the claim, regardless of the present state of the science. Don't expect miracles from a 10. And don't bother with a 2.

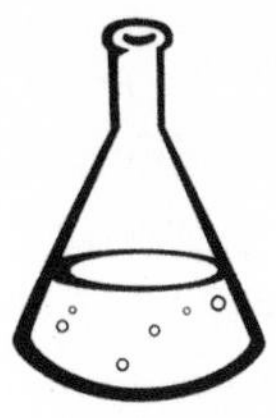

Scientific Validation

There is no black or white when it comes to assessing the quality of research. Studies may produce conflicting results, and ancient remedies that are highly respected elsewhere may not yet have been studied at all. I use my 1-to-20 scale to convey my overall impression of the scientific support. I have relied heavily on the Natural Standard Research Collaboration who specialize in evidence-based information about complementary and alternative therapies. Their assessments of natural medicines reflect the level of available scientific data for or against the use of each therapy for a specific medical condition. So in my ratings, there's no formal support at all for a 0, and a 10 is supported by some evidence but little by way of conclusive studies. A 20 is generally accepted as proven by a consensus of studies. Note that this is different from my personal evaluation of the claim made for the product in column one.

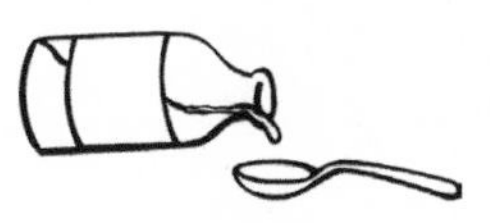

Ease of Compliance

It's no good a remedy being effective if no one's ever going to stick with it. I take into consideration reports back from thousands of patients about taste, format, duration of treatment and availability. A remedy that scores 1 on my scale is very difficult to use or hard to maintain. A 20 is something we can all do.

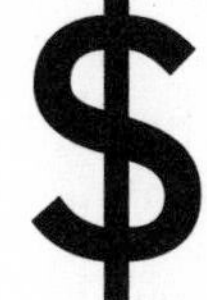

Cost

Because they are "alternative," not all natural or alternative remedies are easily obtained and can therefore be costly. This cost must be weighed against effectiveness. A score of 20 means highly cost-effective, probably less than $1 a day. A low score means more than $5 a day.

Cautions

Alas, as with medications of any sort, no natural remedy is good for everyone all the time. Side effects and possible dangers must be weighed against benefits. I have relied considerably on the Natural Medicines Comprehensive Database (NMCD), the most conservative publication of its kind. A score of 20 means a truly safe remedy. A 10 suggests there is limited evidence but nothing alarming. However, since safety is of paramount importance, the "cautions" score can be a negative number likely to overwhelm all else.

1. THE FIRST DEFENCE: NATURALLY COMBATTING TOXINS, INFECTIONS AND ALLERGENS

In the last chapter, we looked at a wide range of invaders that can threaten our health, and our defences, including our "immunity army." Now let's see what natural products and procedures can be brought onto our side in this noble struggle to maintain health.

CLEANSING AND DETOXIFICATION

There are many things you can do, eat or take to optimize the process by which your body can rid itself of toxins. Think about dealing with trash in your house. The first step is usually to discard it in the waste bin under your sink. The second step is to store it in your garage until collection day. Step three is to place it curbside for the garbage truck to come by to take it away.

Phase I of our body's detoxification process is the first line of defence against all environmental toxins, including pesticides, herbicides, pollutants, solvents, pharmaceuticals and the natural supplements we call nutraceuticals. Specific enzymes take out the garbage for our bodies in every phase. Even naturally occurring chemicals that the body creates (such as waste products and steroid hormones) get detoxified in Phase 1. But as I described in Chapter Two, should there be a mutation in the genes that control for this phase, you could have serious toxicity issues. That's when you could benefit from the realm of available natural medicines to help your body's Phase I detox system work better.

Phase II detoxification follows. Toxins are transformed into water-soluble substances that the body is able to eliminate through the urine or in the feces through the bile. Phase II enzymes of detoxification are involved in what is known as the conjugation or "binding" of toxins, which makes them more extractable from your body. Mutations on the genes governing this process may lead to weight gain, chronic fatigue, headaches and a worsening of virtually any condition for which you are predisposed. Impaired metabolism of the neurotransmitters (dopamine, epinephrine and norepinephrine) that we spoke about in Chapter Two also occurs, and may predispose you to, among many other things, anxiety, ADHD, alcoholism and rapid cycling in bipolar individuals. These mutations can increase or more commonly decrease the activity of our natural detoxification enzymes, but both increased and decreased activity may be harmful. The most important point is reached between Phase I and II, where harmful free radicals are formed as a result of Phase I activity but are transformed to harmless water by antioxidants ingested in our diet. Increased Phase I detoxification without increased detoxification in Phase II can lead to the formation of intermediates that may be more toxic than the original toxin. To use the trash example, you might be great at putting the garbage in the garage, but if you regularly forget to put the trash at the curb, you'll pretty soon be facing a public health issue.

Being an optimal detoxifier requires that from time to time you lend a hand. During these periodic exercises, you help along your liver—the liver is the great detoxification organ—by drinking water and lemon every morning and two or three cups of green tea

To watch a clip about cleansing and natural detoxification support, scan the QR barcode above into your smart device or enter the following link into your browser: http://bit.ly/PBqeEj

per day. You eliminate coffee, alcohol, red meat, pasta/cakes/cookies and other desserts for the duration of a month. You avoid shams such as ionic foot baths and invasive colonics: there isn't any science to support these supposed methods of cleansing. Instead, you incorporate detoxifying foods and natural health products such as red beans, elderberries, cloves, artichokes, mustard, lentils, marjoram, dandelion greens and rosemary, all of which are all excellent detoxifiers. Your supplements including selenium, NAC, glutathione and milk thistle: all of these enhance the liver's ability to clear toxins.

NAC (N-Acetylcysteine)				
			$	!
A respectable detoxifier best known for its work in the ER as an acetaminophen overdose antidote.	Some excellent science in the world of both mainstream and complementary alternative medicine.	It comes in an easy-to-swallow capsule format.	Very affordable.	It is considered safe when used orally, intravenously or inhaled.
18	18	18	18	18
Overall rating: 90%				

COUGHS AND COLDS

Echinacea, a traditional herbal medicine that has been long recognized for its immune-stimulating powers, is the nutraceutical most frequently used in Canada to prevent the common cold. Consumers spend more than $12 million annually on formulas containing echinacea and it is money well spent. Caveat: Be careful to choose a selectively-bred *Echinacea angustifolia* harvested and manufactured following a protocol that causes no immune-suppressive activity. Since this protocol is followed for only a few echinacea products on the market, only a few really work.

To watch a clip about cold and cough support, scan the QR barcode above into your smart device or enter the following link into your browser: http://bit.ly/NQ4kK8

Echinacea *angustifolia* (Jamieson *FluShield*)

When it comes to commonly available products to combat cold and flu viruses, few can compete for sheer visibility with echinacea. This is a name that not many people would have been able to pronounce twenty years ago, yet now it's a favourite for preventing and/or treating colds and flu, right up there with the ginseng compounds and vitamin C.

But if you've heard of echinacea, you've also heard conflicting stories. You have a friend who swears by it. You read somewhere that Native American peoples have relied on it for thousands of years. But someone at work saw a study in the paper that reported it to be useless, of no more value than a placebo. No wonder you're uncertain when you go to the drugstore with those first aches and sniffles. What's the story?

Echinacea typifies the confusion that surrounds the use of many natural health products. These are often plant extracts that have enjoyed long traditional acceptance by one group or another but that have only recently been studied—if it all. The picture is mixed and in a continual state of flux but the direction of change is towards greater and greater understanding.

In the echinacea plant's case, it's not that it's even exotic—the purple coneflower is native to North America and grows easily in the gardens of many of my readers. But that familiarity masks a critical complexity. There are in fact nine species of the plant and only three of these have significant recognized medicinal effects. But what exactly are those effects? And when someone recommends echinacea, what precisely are they recommending? The buds? The flowers? The leaves? The stems? The roots? Because if a user—never mind a study—fails to make these critical distinctions, there's nothing to talk about.

I'd heard a good deal of discussion among professionals about a highly refined echinacea extract that was now widely available through Jamieson, the vitamin company. Jamieson markets the product—FluShield—under licence from the global plant research and development company Indena, a privately owned Italian company with about 800 employees in 70 countries. Some 80 of these employees are engaged in full-time research. Indena was said to have invested twelve years in the research and development of a definitive echinacea product.

In the summer of 2009 I decided to travel to Italy to find out for myself what Jamieson had seen in Indena's work.

Outside the old city of Verona, the company's echinacea plantation stretches all around you. The choice of Verona was no accident: soil and growing conditions were determined to be ideal for the cultivation of the species that Indena's years of research had determined to hold the greatest potential: *Echinecea angustifolia*—the very species that had been widely used by the North American Plains Indians for its general medicinal qualities—and now Polinacea®, the Indena standardized extract from the roots of *Echinacea angustifolia*. Of course it would have been easy to select a growing location in the plant's native North America, but the whole focus of this work was the purity and controllability of the final product. No North American location could be free from the likelihood of cross-pollination by other echinacea species. For added security, Indena uses a system of greenhouse micro-propagation at the Verona facility to make sure that they're growing 100 percent angustifolia.

The medicinally active components of the *Echinacea angustifolia* plant are the alkylamides, the echinacosides and the immunity-enhancing polysaccharides that boost the body's T-cells to fight viral and bacterial invaders. When you buy an echinacea product, it might be made from any part of the plant, but in fact the active compounds are concentrated in the roots. The refinement goes beyond that, however, and illustrates the subtlety of plant extract chemistry.

When echinacosides enter the body, they have little effect on immunity and the alkylamides can actually act to suppress immune system activity. At the Indena production facilities in Milan, the levels of these components are significantly lowered and the polysaccharides concentrated and tightly standardized. Such precision is generally associated with the pharmaceutical industry, but we're seeing it increasingly applied to natural extracts. This is what is meant by the term "nutraceutical." At any rate, the proof of the pudding is in the eating: the Indena echinacea product, the raw material from which Jamieson goes on to produce FluShield, has been clinically proven to reduce the symptoms of colds and flu when taken in the early stages.

The study and refinement of plant materials to produce effective natural health products is only getting under way. You can't expect everything on the shelves of your neighbourhood pharmacy to have the benefit of the intense and expensive research and development that has gone into FluShield and related products. But the picture is changing—and improving—every year.

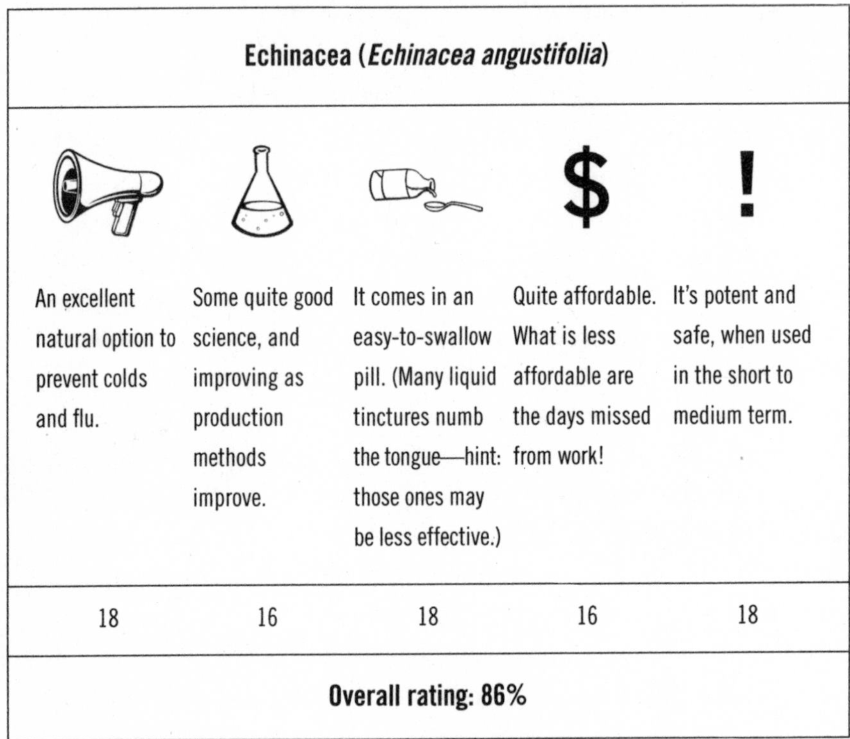

Echinacea (*Echinacea angustifolia*)				
An excellent natural option to prevent colds and flu.	Some quite good science, and improving as production methods improve.	It comes in an easy-to-swallow pill. (Many liquid tinctures numb the tongue—hint: those ones may be less effective.)	Quite affordable. What is less affordable are the days missed from work!	It's potent and safe, when used in the short to medium term.
18	16	18	16	18
Overall rating: 86%				

Andrographis is a herbal remedy that has been widely used in Indian and Ayurvedic forms of medicine for upper respiratory tract infections. A combination of andrographis with Siberian ginseng (*Eleutherococcus senticosus*, not related to ordinary ginseng but long recognized in traditional Chinese medicine; also called "eleuthero") can be effective for the treatment of upper respiratory tract infections. In a clinical study, this mixture was administered for five days and was shown to improve fever, sore throat and cough.

Andrographis (*Andrographis paniculata*)				
A very powerful herb for upper respiratory infections.	This herb gets an A for science.	It comes in many formats but is quite bitter in tincture form.	Quite affordable.	This herb has less than a handful of reports of major allergic reactions. "Likely Safe" (NMCD).
18	18	16	16	18
Overall rating: 86%				

Goldenseal, or *Hydrastis canadensis*, is nature's antibiotic. I've seen it work wonders both personally and in my practice. Goldenseal is a popular treatment for the common cold and upper respiratory tract infections that lead to coughs. It is likely that the active goldenseal component, berberine, has effects against bacteria and inflammation.

However, it doesn't have a perfect track record.

Goldenseal (*Hydrastis canadensis*)				
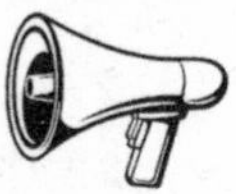	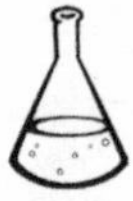	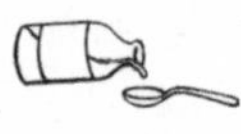	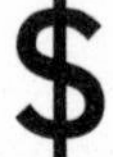	!
To kick a bad upper respiratory infection, it's your best friend!	Not yet supported by the strongest science.	Due to its pungent taste, it is often reported as very difficult to swallow in liquid or powder form.	One of the more expensive herbs.	Where goldenseal is potent, it does have a few heart, skin, stomach, liver and nervous system warnings when taken at high doses. Caution is warranted.
18	14	10	14	10
Overall rating: 66%				

SUPPORTING OUR IMMUNITY ARMY

If you are the type of person who is always getting sick or coming down with the latest viral infection, immune-boosting strategies may be for you. And for those of you who think you're really healthy, good health is no guarantee that you'll never get sick. It will, however, influence how you manage the illness. If your immune system has never encountered a particular virus or bacteria in the past, you'll likely become infected. If you're exceptionally healthy, that may only translate into a briefly elevated temperature, a day's worth of aches and pains, and temporary symptoms related to infection. If you have an unhealthy constitution, you may experience long-drawn-out symptoms and bacterial complications.

To watch a clip about immune support, scan the QR barcode above into your smart device or enter the following link into your browser: http://bit.ly/PBBKj3

The same natural health products that are effective for coughs and colds can provide the general logistical support our immunity army needs if it's to remain numerous, active and powerful. *Echinacea angustifolia* helps to significantly boost activity of the immune system. For more than two thousand years, the roots of ginseng have been valued in Chinese medicine, and may be an effective agent for immune system enhancement. Probiotics are beneficial bacteria—sometimes called the "friendly germs"—that help maintain a healthy intestine, where it is believed that about 80 percent of our immune system lives. Lastly, zinc appears to be an essential trace element for the immune system because it improves white blood cell counts *and* activity. Talk to a professional about what doses and duration may be right for *you*.

THE WAR AGAINST THE GERMS: SUMMONING OUR NATURAL ALLIES

Natural health products can play an important role in slowing the development of methicillin-resistant *Staphylococcus aureus* (or MRSA) and similar bacteria. Rather than throwing powerful antibiotics at nearly everything that presents as an infection—including viral infections, which are not affected by antibiotics—we can use antibacterial and antiseptic herbs, homeopathics and nutraceuticals as a first line of defence.

Topically, iodine has been used for many years as a disinfectant for cleaning wounds, sterilizing skin before surgical or invasive procedures, or sterilizing catheter entry sites.

Some excellent modern research shows that probiotics—the same beneficial bacteria we mentioned when discussing the reinforcement of our immune system—help maintain a healthy intestine by keeping harmful bacteria and yeasts in the gut under control. Probiotics can be taken as capsules, tablets, beverages, powders, yogurts and other foods. An increasing number of studies support the use of probiotics as a supplement to antibiotic therapy. Some probiotics may also help prevent the development of antibiotic resistance and evidence with daycare children given probiotics suggests a reduction in the number of sick days, the frequency of respiratory tract infections and the frequency of related antibiotic treatments.

Probiotics (*Bifidobacterium, Lactobacillus, Saccharomyces boulardii*)				
			$	!
If your gut says you have an issue, treat it with probiotics!	Excellent and rapidly growing science to support broad use of probiotics	Easy and pleasant to take in yogurt, powder and pill form	Moderately expensive—usually more than $3/day	"Likely safe" (NMCD)
18	18	16	14	14
Overall rating: 80%				

Finally, botanicals such as astragalus (derived from the roots of *Astragalus membranaceus*, native to China) and goldenseal

(*Hydrastis canadensis*) possess strong antimicrobial properties and are therefore effective against bacterial infection.

To watch a clip about infection and antiseptic support, scan the QR barcode above into your smart device or enter the following link into your browser: http://bit.ly/MAW1V8

HELP WITH YEAST INFECTIONS

If a woman supplements her diet with probiotics, it may prevent the overgrowth of yeast organisms called vaginitis. If an infection does appear, placing a small amount of yogurt intravaginally before bed can help or, if the infection is stubborn, boric acid capsules inserted intravaginally have been used successfully as a treatment.

To watch a clip about yeast infection support, scan the QR barcode above into your smart device or enter the following link into your browser: http://bit.ly/M6qzjA

SUPPORT FOR THE URINARY TRACT

Cranberry juice is a well-known natural treatment for urinary tract infections. You might find the reasons for its effectiveness interesting. Most UTIs are caused by the bacteria *E. coli,* which can attach themselves to the lining of the urinary tract by binding to molecules of mannose that naturally occur there. Peaches, oranges, apples and certain berries, including cranberries and blueberries, contain large amounts of a sugar called D-mannose, which is poorly absorbed by the body and ends up in the bloodstream and hence the urine. The D-mannose molecules make it difficult for the bacteria to attach to the mannose molecules on the surfaces of the urinary system.

If it's been determined that you have an *E. coli* infection, you can treat it and prevent recurrences by drinking 4 to 10 ounces of cranberry juice a day, or taking 400 mg of powdered cranberry concentrate twice a day. Goldenseal (*Hydrastis canadensis L.*) contains berberine, an alkaloid that may prevent certain UTIs through a mechanism similar to that of cranberry juice. Although it doesn't yet have any powerhouse science to back it up, this is another natural remedy to consider.

To watch a clip about urinary tract infection support, scan the QR barcode above into your smart device or enter the following link into your browser: http://bit.ly/OcPkbO

You may be surprised to hear that if and when you need to take antiobiotics, you may be able to enhance their effectiveness by taking proteolytic enzymes such as bromelain and trypsin along with them. If you don't really have symptoms of a urinary tract infection, or it is rare or unusual for you to have one, ask your doctor to send your urine for culture and not to rely on an on-site "urine chemistry" test. And, remember that antibiotics can't tell the good intestinal flora from the bad, so recharge your digestive system with *pro*biotics after the *anti*biotic treatment is complete.

DEALING WITH ALLERGIES

If testing indicates that you suffer from environmental allergies, you can find relief through a number of natural health products.

First, consider increasing your nutritional intake of omega-3 fatty acids and brightly coloured fruits and vegetables that contain flavonoids. (If you know you have an allergy to any of them, ask your doctor if you can stew your fruits, as this practice will usually remove the allergens). To help you further, you might want to try spirulina, a type of blue-green algae available as a supplement that may act to decrease the symptoms of allergies.

The perennial shrub butterbur may prevent symptoms from allergies. In fact, comparisons of butterbur to prescription drugs have reported similar efficacy. I recommend a herbal extract standardized to contain 8 mg of petasin (a butterbur extract) per tablet taken two or three times a day for two weeks. Caution: the raw, unprocessed plant is potentially toxic and you should avoid butterbur if you are allergic or hypersensitive to plants from the Asteraceae or Compositae family such as ragweed, marigolds, daisies and chrysanthemums.

To watch a clip about the neti pot, scan the QR barcode above into your smart device or enter the following link into your browser: http://bit.ly/MEMZZh

Homeopathic sublingual immunotherapy—oral treatment using dilute amounts of the allergen itself also known as SLIT—can result in better overall tolerance of allergies. And did you know that effective allergy prevention should include showering your nose? Nasal irrigation, using a "neti pot," effectively treats allergies and chronic sinusitis.

Essentially, you prepare a warm, saltwater solution in a special ceramic pot known as a neti pot and pour it through your nose to relieve your sinuses and rinse away the nagging allergens, dust and bacteria. And don't forget to shower the rest of you—especially your hair and especially before bedtime—to wash out the allergens that may be stuck to your skin. Wash clothes in hot water—this destroys allergens—and consider the use of a high-efficiency particulate air (HEPA) purifier to clean the circulating

To watch a clip about allergy support, scan the QR barcode above into your smart device or enter the following link into your browser: http://bit.ly/Oinhpy

air. You might also consider a dehumidifier to reduce dust mites and fungi.

SINUS SUFFERING

If you suffer from chronic sinus congestion, you can breathe freely again by clearing the blocked passageways and thus easing the sinus pressure. First, keep your environment free of irritants and allergens such as dust, mould, smoke, chemical fumes and animal dander that can trigger sinus congestion. Then try "steam cleaning" your sinuses with aromatic oils such as eucalyptus or products containing menthol: this should reduce nasal stuffiness. Nasal irrigation also works well, using the method described above for dealing with allergies. Also, don't overlook the possibility of food allergies when you have sinus symptoms. Work with a knowledgeable practitioner to find out if food allergens may contribute to your congestion.

Bromelain, the digestive enzyme that is extracted from the stem and the fruit of the pineapple plant, has been studied for its effects on sinusitis, and a 2007 German study found that a herbal mixture of nasturtium and horseradish may be comparable to antibiotics for the treatment of acute sinusitis. Good scientific evidence suggests butterbur (*Petasites hybridus*) is effective for the prevention of allergic rhinitis in susceptible individuals and may also prevent chronic bacterial sinusitis that can be a secondary consequence of allergies.

To watch a clip about sinus support, scan the QR barcode above into your smart device or enter the following link into your browser: http://bit.ly/NHc1DX

Use of the probiotic *Enterococcus faecalis* bacteria for sinus inflammation may reduce the frequency of relapses and the need for antibiotic therapy.

Butterbur (*Petasites hybridus*)				
An allergy miracle!	The science backing butterbur easily stands up to conventional remedies.	Easy to take in capsule form.	Affordable at about $2/day.	"Possibly safe" (NMCD).
18	16	18	16	10
Overall rating: 78%				

2. WHAT GOES IN:NATURAL SUPPORT FOR DIET AND DIGESTION

Digestion is a huge subject and there's a huge volume of traditional and modern remedies, natural and otherwise. Here are my suggestions for some of the best—and the rest. But if I had to give one piece of advice to cover all, it would be: "Bodies, not factories, should process food."

RELIEF FROM INDIGESTION

It may surprise you to learn that heartburn and indigestion may be caused by too *little* stomach acid. This may seem to be a paradox, but based on my clinical experience, supplementing with a natural health product like betaine HCl (a compound that *contains* hydrochloric acid) often relieves the symptoms of heartburn and improves digestion.

It is important to realize that when you experience indigestion, your vitamin absorption may be compromised. Many minerals and vitamins—iron, zinc and B-complex vitamins including folic acid—appear to require adequate concentrations of stomach acid to be absorbed optimally.

To watch a clip about digestion support, scan the QR barcode above into your smart device or enter the following link into your browser: http://bit.ly/OcbsCW

There are many natural health products that may improve general digestion. Some very effective ones derive from caraway, the popular culinary spice. Aside from its cooking uses, the volatile oil from the seeds is effective in managing heartburn, bloating, cramping and abdominal pain. I also recommend it to patients with chronic problems such as irritable bowel syndrome and acid reflux.

Other natural health products proven to optimize digestion are probiotics—the "good bacteria"—enteric-coated peppermint oil, artichoke, ginger and of course digestive enzymes, such as a broad-spectrum combination protease, lipase and amylase.

RELIEF FOR THE GUT

Constipation and indigestion. You've seen your health-care practitioners but nothing sinister is suspected. What can you do apart from relying on commercial pharmaceuticals?

To begin, try a bulk laxative. For results within 12 to 24 hours, take 5 to 10 grams per day of psyllium husk or 3 to 4 grams per day of glucomannan mixed in water, followed by a second glass of water. Psyllium is derived from the husks of the seeds of *Plantago ovata* and contains a high level of soluble dietary fibre. It's the chief ingredient in many commonly used bulk laxatives. Most studies of psyllium report an increase in stool weight, an increase in bowel movements per day and a decrease in total gut transit time.

Next, increase your fruits and veggies and get more fibre and water in your diet. Include more beans, bran, flaxseed and whole grains in your diet. Phosphates are the naturally occurring form of the element phosphorus and as a laxative, phosphates appear to increase peristalsis (movement of the gastrointestinal tract) and cause an entry of fluids into the intestine. Similarly, the calcium-magnesium balance of the body is critically important for cellular function and magnesium deficiency commonly leads to constipation. Supplementing with magnesium glycinate 100 mg daily not only improves bowel regularity but has been shown to lengthen telomeres.

The inner lining of aloe leaves, taken by mouth, has been used traditionally as a laxative and the laxative properties of aloe components such as aloin are well supported by scientific evidence.

Aloe (*Aloe Vera*)				
Got constipation? A skin ailment? A sunburn? Aloe to the rescue!	The efficacy of aloe is supported by a considerable number of studies.	Easy to take in liquid form. A mild and pleasant taste. Widely available.	Very affordable at about $1/day.	"Likely Safe to Possibly safe" (NMCD).
18	16	18	18	17
Overall rating: 87%				

Flaxseed is a mild, bulk-forming laxative that's best suited for long-term use in people with constipation.

Lastly, let's not forget our old friends the probiotics. Taking them as a supplement will help maintain a population of healthy intestinal flora. An insufficiency of these digestive allies can cause either constipation or diarrhea.

RELIEF FROM INFANTILE COLIC

Some research has suggested that certain natural health products containing fennel, chamomile and lemon balm are potential treatments for breastfed colic in infants. More recent research done at Regina Margherita Children's Hospital in Italy suggests that daily probiotics may improve symptoms associated with infantile colic. The Italian researchers concluded that the probiotic *L. reuteri* may improve colicky symptoms in breastfed infants within one week of treatment. This compared favourably with simethicone, an oral anti-foaming agent commonly used to reduce bloating, discomfort and pain caused by excess gas in the stomach or intestinal tract.

Because homeopathy is safe and effective for infants and children, it too is commonly a solution for colic. The remedy *carbo vegetabilis* releases intestinal gas often related to abdominal discomfort; *colocynthis* can relax cramping of the intestinal tract and *cuprum metallicum* relaxes spasms of the abdominal area. Any and all of these homeopathic remedies offer your baby relief and comfort and can afford *you* a good night's sleep.

To watch a clip about colic support, scan the QR barcode above into your smart device or enter the following link into your browser: http://bit.ly/PBrDuL

COPING WITH IRRITABLE BOWEL SYNDROME

Irritable bowel syndrome (IBS) is a relatively common gastrointestinal disorder that causes significant discomfort. The cause of IBS remains unknown, but recent research suggests a brain-gut connection. IBS is not related to inflammatory bowel diseases, such as Crohn's disease or ulcerative colitis (see below). Common symptoms include abdominal bloating, gas, diarrhea and/or constipation. Research shows that people with IBS are more likely than others to have backaches, fatigue and several other seemingly unrelated problems.

If you suffer from IBS, the first remedy is to consume the right fibre. Examples are fibre-rich flaxseed, rye, brown rice, oatmeal, barley and vegetables. Sometimes IBS sufferers improve as a result of taking a bulk-forming laxative such as psyllium husk. It *is* necessary to strike a balance between the amount of fibre to ensure regularity and not getting so much as to trigger episodes of diarrhea.

Exploring food sensitivities is one of the most effective approaches to resolving the underlying cause of IBS. Work with a specialist to identify foods that aggravate your condition. This often requires experimentally removing gluten, dairy products, corn, beans, foods containing caffeine, fructose and sorbitol from your diet.

Peppermint and caraway oils can effectively manage symptoms for some sufferers. Taking a coated herbal supplement providing 0.2 to 0.4 ml of peppermint oil, preferably combined with 50 mg of caraway oil, three times a day may reduce gas production, ease intestinal cramping and soothe the intestinal tract.

COPING WITH CELIAC DISEASE

Celiac disease is an intestinal disorder that results from an abnormal immune reaction to gluten, a protein found in wheat, barley, rye and, to a lesser extent, oats. Surprisingly, about one in a hundred people has celiac and of those who do a staggering 97 percent don't know it!

Celiac disease can affect other parts of the body, such as the pancreas (increasing the risk of diabetes), the thyroid gland (increasing the risk of thyroid disease) and the nervous system (increasing the risk of peripheral neuropathies and other neurological disorders). It is also commonly associated with a chronic skin disorder called dermatitis herpetiformis. Occasionally, damage occurs in one or more of these parts of the body in the *absence* of damage to the intestines. In a certain few, celiac may not cause symptoms at all. However, others may have a history of frequent diarrhea; pale, foul-smelling, bulky stools; abdominal pain, gas and bloating; weight loss; fatigue; canker sores; muscle cramps; delayed growth or short stature; bone and joint pain; seizures; painful skin rash; or even infertility.

Obviously, once testing has confirmed celiac, the best treatment is avoidance of gluten, and the present-day marketplace is rich in gluten-free products: breads, flours and cereals. Since the malabsorption that occurs in celiac disease can lead to multiple nutritional deficiencies, supplementing with a broad-spectrum multivitamin and mineral may help to correct a deficiency. The best solution to discover nutrient deficiency—celiac or not—is a comprehensive blood, urine and hair tissue analysis for micronutrient deficiencies.

CROHN'S DISEASE AND ULCERATIVE COLITIS

Crohn's disease is a poorly understood inflammatory condition that usually affects the ileo-cecal area (the lower part of the small intestine) and the beginning and midsection of the colon. The most common symptoms during flare-ups include bloody stools, malabsorption problems, chronic diarrhea with abdominal pain, occasional fever, loss of appetite, weight loss and a sense of fullness in the abdomen. About one-third of people with Crohn's have a history of anal fissures or fistulas.

A variety of probiotic preparations have shown effectiveness in preventing relapse or maintaining remission in Crohn's. There is also limited but promising research of the use of oral aloe vera in ulcerative colitis.

Fish oil helps relieve the inflammation of the gut that occurs in people suffering from Crohn's disease, while bovine colostrum and chlorella may improve gastrointestinal health and may be an effective treatment in gut inflammation and general immune function.

It is important to note that malabsorption is common in Crohn's and can lead to a deficiency in many vitamins, including vitamin D. Supplementing with it can help prevent bone loss in cases of deficiency but also support the immune system.

To watch a clip about Crohn's disease support, scan the QR barcode above into your smart device or enter the following link into your browser: http://bit.ly/LIFMBf

Worth noting: in one small trial, six of seven people with Crohn's disease went into remission after taking DHEA (dehydroepiandrosterone) for eight weeks.

DEALING WITH LACTOSE INTOLERANCE

To remedy lactose intolerance, over-the-counter products containing lactase enzyme can be supplemented when consuming foods containing lactose.

An interesting new study suggests that supplementation of infant formulas with probiotics is one approach for the management of cow's milk allergy. Probiotics have been found to enhance the digestion and absorption of proteins, fats, calcium and phosphorus. It may also turn out that they can help to overcome lactose intolerance.

If you are among those people who need to avoid dairy, you should consider a calcium supplement providing 500 to 1,000 mg per day.

To watch a clip about lactose intolerance, scan the QR barcode above into your smart device or enter the following link into your browser: http://bit.ly/NNlaMt

To watch a clip about leaky gut support, scan the QR barcode above into your smart device or enter the following link into your browser: http://bit.ly/MjCtBS

HEALING THE LEAKY GUT

If, as I believe, leaky gut syndrome contributes to intestinal dysfunction, I have several recommendations to help you achieve optimal intestinal health. Aside from a healthy diet—one that also avoids foods you are allergic to or sensitive to—and the avoidance of the bad habits I just mentioned, I recommend natural health products that can help reverse this syndrome. Examples are the bioactive proteins such as lactoperoxidase lactoferrin, globulin proteins, arabinogalactans and fructooligosaccharides. All support the growth of health-supporting bacteria. Meanwhile, phosphatidylcholine, L-glutamine and licorice protect and nourish the intestinal lining. Finally, high doses of broad-spectrum supplemental probiotics appear to be strongly supportive of intestinal health.

L-Glutamine (*2,5-Diamino-5-oxopentaenoic acid*)				
			$	!
Good gut-healing potential, used by weight trainers to increase muscle. Amazing for burn victims.	Well-designed studies support the use of glutamine as part of an intravenous nutrition protocol in postsurgical, burn or wasting patients, Further research in patients with malnutrition, digestive concerns or other illnesses is warranted.	Easy to take in powder form. Best mixed into juice.	Affordable at about $2/day.	"Possibly safe" (NMCD).
16	14	18	16	10
Overall rating: 74%				

SUPPORTING THE LIVER

Because of the many roles it plays in maintaining our body's functions, the liver deserves special mention, whether you're diagnosed as having a liver problem or not. In order to remain healthy, your body requires an optimally functioning liver to deal with the food you eat, the hormones and metabolites that your body naturally produces, and your inevitable exposure to toxins. To date, some of the best studied natural health products to support the liver are milk thistle extracts, betaine and cordyceps.

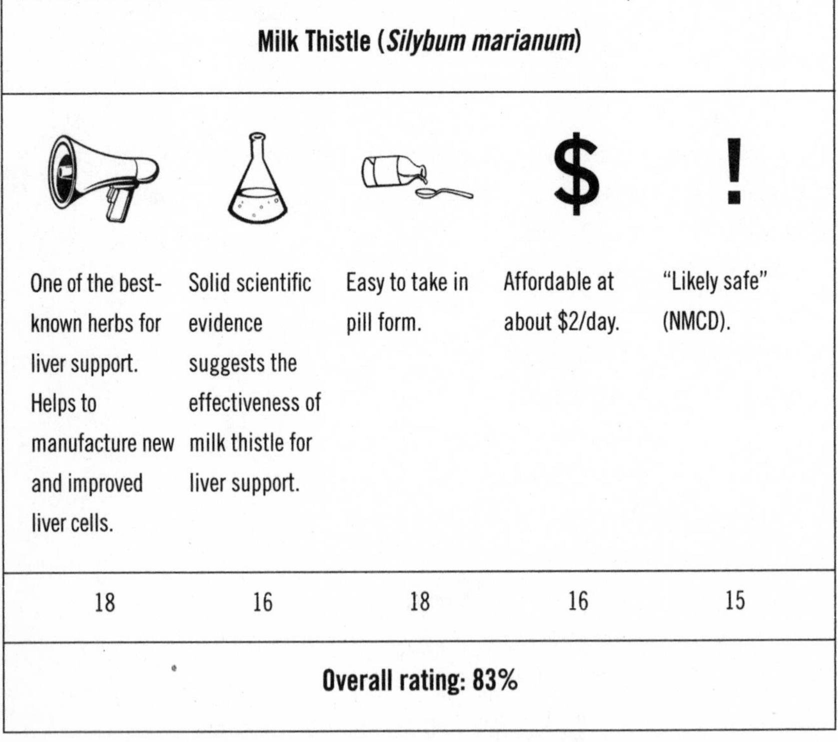

Milk Thistle (*Silybum marianum*)				
			$	!
One of the best-known herbs for liver support. Helps to manufacture new and improved liver cells.	Solid scientific evidence suggests the effectiveness of milk thistle for liver support.	Easy to take in pill form.	Affordable at about $2/day.	"Likely safe" (NMCD).
18	16	18	16	15
Overall rating: 83%				

Multiple studies suggest the benefits of oral milk thistle using the flavonoid complex called silymarin extracted from the seeds of milk thistle. Milk thistle is commonly grown throughout

North America and Europe and has found application as a medicinal agent for more than two thousand years, principally for disorders of the liver and gallbladder.

In experiments lasting up to five years, milk thistle improved liver function and even decreased the number of deaths that occur in people with cirrhosis. Several studies of oral milk thistle for chronic hepatitis caused by viruses or alcohol have shown improvements in liver function tests.

To watch a clip about liver support, scan the QR barcode above into your smart device or enter the following link into your browser: http://bit.ly/NH6Zr2

Betaine is found in most microorganisms, plants, marine animals and many foods, especially beets, spinach, grain and shellfish. Its main physiological functions are to protect cells under stress.

Traditional Chinese medicine has used cordyceps to support and improve liver function. It's known to stimulate the immune system and may improve serum gamma globulin levels in people with hepatitis B.

THE CARE AND FEEDING OF THE PEPTIC ULCER

You probably won't understand the importance of preventing a peptic ulcer until you have one. As we know, *H. pylori* is the prime suspect, yet there are other factors that may either directly cause ulcers or encourage the growth of a helicobacter infection. Whatever the cause, when an ulcer happens, your concern will be the healing process.

Start by avoiding irritants—in particular, smoking, aspirin and related drugs, alcohol, coffee (including decaf), tea and hot spices. All can aggravate an ulcer. Reduce the risk of new and recurrent duodenal ulcers by getting enough fibre.

To watch a clip about ulcer support, scan the QR barcode above into your smart device or enter the following link into your browser: http://bit.ly/NsjmtX

One of the most effective natural health products for ulcers is zinc. This mineral and its bound counterpart, zinc-carnosine, are known to speed the repair of damaged tissue in the digestive lining.

Deglycerized licorice root (DGL) has a long history of use for soothing inflamed and injured mucous membranes in the digestive tract. Flavonoids in licorice may also inhibit growth of *H. pylori.*

DGL (*deglycyrrhizinated licorice*)				
Fast-acting heartburn remedy.	Moderate scientific support.	Easy to take in chewable-tablet form.	Affordable at about $2/day .	"Possibly safe" (NMCD).
18	14	18	16	12
Overall rating: 78%				

Mastic, the gummy extract of *Pistachia lentiscus*, also known as mastic gum, has been shown in studies to heal peptic ulcers.

Ayurvedic doctors in India have traditionally used dried banana powder to treat ulcers. Banana powder appears to protect the lining of the stomach from acid. Ayurvedic medicine also found an important role for the extracts of the neem tree (*Azadirachta indica*) of India and Burma. Such extracts are traditionally credited with a reduction in stomach acid levels and near-complete healing of people with duodenal ulcers.

GETTING UNSTONED

Researchers haven't as yet established a clear relationship between diet and gallstone formation but the evidence points towards low-fibre, high-cholesterol diets and diets high in starchy foods as being causative factors. Obese women have seven times the risk of forming gallstones compared with women who are not overweight. Even slightly overweight women have significantly higher risks and this suggests a regular exercise program and generally keeping fit and trim will reduce your risk. Oddly though, *rapid* weight loss actually appears to increase the risk. Other risk factors are constipation, eating a small number of meals per day, low fish consumption and low intake of the nutrients folate, magnesium, calcium and vitamin C. This may explain why some studies suggest wine and whole-grain bread may decrease the risk of gallstones. (Actually, it doesn't explain why a bit of wine helps—but who cares, if it's something you enjoy!) Certainly wheat bran—two tablespoons a day of unprocessed wheat bran with plenty of liquid—can decrease cholesterol build-up.

If you're a vegetarian, it seems to be good news for your gallbladder. A low-fat diet rich in vegetables, beans and other vegetarian foods has shown benefits against gallstone formation. Uncovering food allergies can also help.

Liver flushing is an alternative method purported to remove gallstones, which accumulate in the gallbladder and/or liver. Flushing involves drinking a concoction of olive oil, epsom salts, soda and lemon juice at night at intervals along with a coffee enema. The diarrhea so produced is said to force out many

To watch a clip about gallstone support, scan the QR barcode above into your smart device or enter the following link into your browser: http://bit.ly/MXcRtb

gallstones. Do *not* try this if you have what your doctor tells you are "large" gallstones—the kind that won't fit through the common bile duct. If you do, this practice could send you to the hospital in a hurry by lodging one and forcing the emergency removal of your gallbladder.

Apart from exercise and good nutrition, there are some effective natural health products to help prevent or treat gallstones. It's always heartening when extracts from vegetables and good scientific studies come together, as they have recently to demonstrate that globe artichoke extract works as a choleretic, increasing bile secretion from the gallbladder. Globe artichoke is one of the world's oldest recognized medicinal plants.

In a study undertaken by the University of Kentucky Medical Center, Brigham and Women's Hospital, and Harvard Medical School, it was shown that magnesium consumption may have a role in the prevention of symptomatic gallstone disease among men. This is one more endorsement for magnesium, an abundant element in the human body and known to be involved in 300 enzymatic reactions therein.

Phosphatidycholine—a major component of lecithin—has received some support from research for treatment of hepatitis and the body's defence system. According to some theories, it may also help dissolve gallstones and prevent them from recurring.

KIDNEY STONES

If your doctor confirms that you suffer from the common calcium oxalate kidney stone—or you have suffered from such stones, even though they're now gone—you'll want to prevent a recurrence. Kidney stones are highly associated with metabolic syndrome and excess body fat percentage.

Reduction of body fat and drinking plenty of fluids are the first steps in prevention. Water, lemonade and most fruit juices can help dilute the substances in the urine that form kidney stones. Avoid soft drinks, especially colas, which contain phosphoric acid, a stone inducer. Avoiding grapefruit juice may also help. The research as to why grapefruit juice increases the risk of kidney stones is inconclusive. However, some research shows that people who consumed 8 ounces of grapefruit juice every day increased their chances of developing kidney stones by 44 percent during a period of eight years.

Diets high in animal protein are linked to increased calcium in the urine, which contributes to oxalate stones. This is also, of course, preventative for gallstones. Avoid foods rich in organic acids (oxalates) that help stones form. That means limiting spinach, rhubarb, beetroot greens, nuts, chocolate, tea, bran, almonds, peanuts and strawberries, which appear to increase urinary oxalate levels.

Supplementing with 50 mg a day of vitamin B6 and 200 to 400 mg a day of magnesium (preferably the citrate form) may inhibit oxalate stone formation. A combination of potassium citrate and magnesium citrate may also reduce the recurrence rate; IP-6 or inositol hexaphosphate, also called phytic acid, reduces urinary calcium levels and may reduce the risk of forming a kidney stone. Even if you can't adhere totally to such a regimen, everything you do along these lines may help prevent a recurrence. If you've ever had kidney stones, you know it will be worth it.

To watch a clip about kidney support, scan the QR barcode above into your smart device or enter the following link into your browser: http://bit.ly/OjP3BX

3. SEXUAL HEALING: NATURAL HEALTH FOR WOMEN AND MEN

I see lots of patients with problems related to sexuality and reproduction and get lots of questions from the public on these issues. But surprisingly, relatively few people think of natural health products in this connection. Let me offer a sampling by way of demonstrating that most people underestimate the potential help available.

WOMEN'S HEALTH

PMS Support

Premenstrual syndrome or PMS is a poorly understood complex of symptoms, occurring a week to ten days before the start of each menstrual cycle, and is believed to be triggered by changes in progesterone and estrogen levels. Symptoms include cramping, bloating, mood changes and breast tenderness.

Women with PMS who jogged an average of about twelve miles a week for six months were reported to experience a reduction in breast tenderness, fluid retention, depression and stress.

It has long been known that vitamin B6 can be helpful in managing PMS. But a new study suggests that women who simply maintain a diet rich in overall B vitamins may have a reduced risk of PMS. According to this study, B vitamins—including thiamine, riboflavin, niacin, vitamin B6, folate and vitamin B12—are required to create brain chemicals that may play a role in alleviating PMS. The researchers found that women who consumed high quantities of riboflavin (vitamin B2) and thiamine (vitamin B1) in particular had a much lower risk of developing PMS.

Recent research also suggests that a combination of essential fatty acids and vitamin E may help to reduce PMS symptoms. Another new study has suggested that St. John's wort plus Vitex may be beneficial.

Calcium and magnesium are important in helping to reduce mood swings, bloating, headaches and other PMS symptoms. L-tryptophan or even 5-HTP during the second half of the menstrual cycle may help balance mood symptoms.

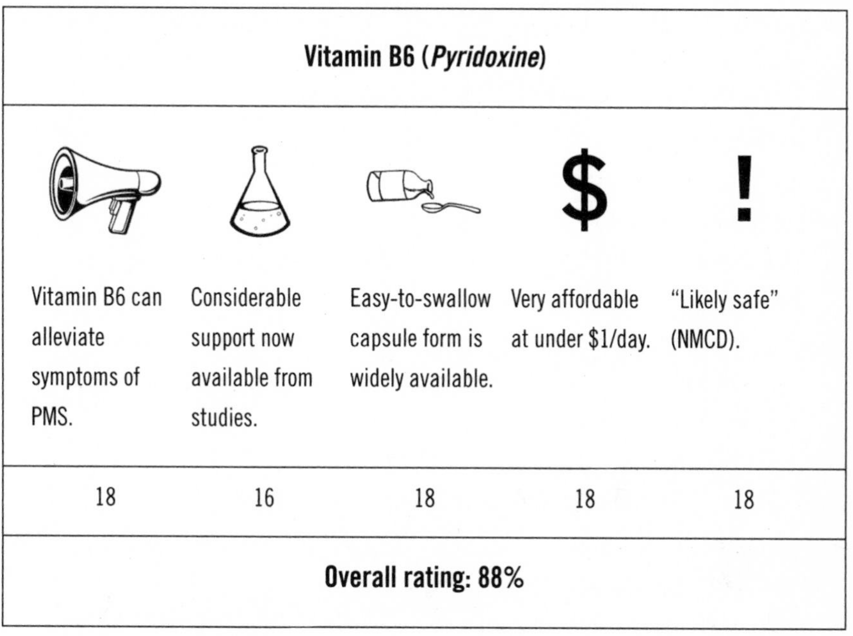

Vitamin B6 (*Pyridoxine*)				
Vitamin B6 can alleviate symptoms of PMS.	Considerable support now available from studies.	Easy-to-swallow capsule form is widely available.	Very affordable at under $1/day.	"Likely safe" (NMCD).
18	16	18	18	18
Overall rating: 88%				

Natural Breast Health

There are many natural health products that may support breast health. Here are a few that I feel deserve your attention.

Bilberry, a close relative of the blueberry, has a long history of medicinal use. Some research suggests that it may be beneficial in the treatment of fibrocystic breast disease.

Black cohosh (*Cimicifuga racemosa* or *Actaea racemosa*) is a member of the buttercup family and an immensely popular remedy for hormone-related symptoms including pre- and post-menopausal symptoms such as hot flashes and irritability. Based on this widespread use, a 2007 study found some evidence that

To watch a clip about breast health support, scan the QR barcode above into your smart device or enter the following link into your browser: http://bit.ly/SQB4qi

black cohosh appears to be associated with a *protective* effect for breast cancer.

The chasteberry tree (*Vitex agnus-castus*) is native to the Mediterranean and Central Asia. Its berries have long been used for a variety of abnormalities including breast pain and menstrual abnormalities.

Lastly, evening primrose oil (*Oenothera biennis L.*) contains an omega-6 essential fatty acid, gamma-linolenic acid (GLA), which is believed to be the active ingredient. Evening primrose oil may have an effect on treating breast cysts and is commonly used for breast pain.

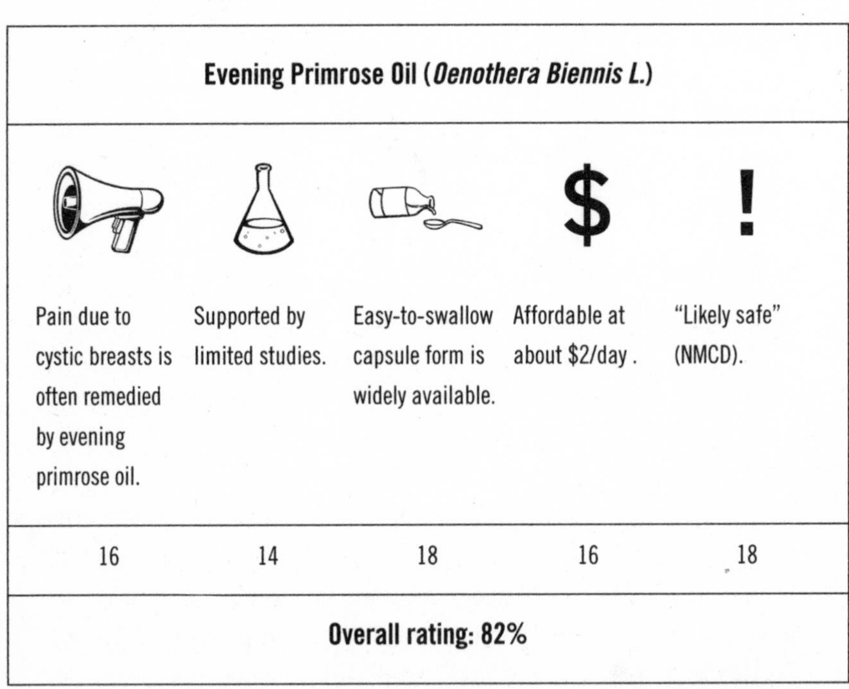

Evening Primrose Oil (*Oenothera Biennis L.*)				
Pain due to cystic breasts is often remedied by evening primrose oil.	Supported by limited studies.	Easy-to-swallow capsule form is widely available.	Affordable at about $2/day .	"Likely safe" (NMCD).
16	14	18	16	18
Overall rating: 82%				

Pregnancy

Every pregnant woman wants to do whatever she can to ensure the optimal health and vitality of her baby. Natural health products including essential vitamins and minerals can play a vital role to improving the health of your unborn child, but you must *always* check with your doctor before taking anything, whether promoted as natural, sold over the counter, or obtained otherwise.

To watch a clip about pregnancy support, scan the QR barcode above into your smart device or enter the following link into your browser: http://bit.ly/MjG5Uw

Fact: taking a multivitamin three months prior to and three months into a pregnancy has been associated with a reduced rate of many birth defects.

Omega-3 fatty acids are probably the most important supplement you can take while pregnant. The omega-3 fatty acid DHA is especially important for fetal and childhood development. During pregnancy, large amounts of DHA and arachidonic acid, commonly found in fish oil, are deposited in the fetal eye and brain and seem to be critical for normal nervous system and visual development. Babies with the highest levels of the omega-3 fatty acids in cord blood had the best hand–eye coordination and when assessed later in life performed better in all areas of development, including personal, social, speech and hearing, performance, and practical reasoning. They also had higher scores for receptive language, average phrase length and vocabulary. In fact, many authorities believe that a child's IQ may increase as a consequence of having received prenatal fish oil.

Other studies show *postnatal* supplementation with fish oil increases IQ. A clinical study conducted on 175 four-year-old preschool children, randomly chosen from eleven different sites in the United States, confirmed that regular intake of fish oil—specifically

To watch a clip about omega-3 essential fatty acids, scan the QR barcode above into your smart device or enter the following link into your browser: http://bit.ly/MXakPG

DHA—boosts intelligence in children. It confirmed that the intake of 400 mg of docoxahexaenoic acid (DHA) caused a rise in DHA levels in the blood of children by up to 300 percent. The study also analyzed the relationship of this rise to the children's performance on a Peabody Picture Vocabulary Test, which measures listening, comprehension and vocabulary. They found that for every 1 percent increase in blood DHA in the children, percentile rank on their PPV test improved by up to nine points.

Another study published in the *American Journal of Clinical Nutrition* showed that people who eat oily fish or take fish oil supplements score 13 percent higher in IQ tests and are prone to healthier brain aging.

Folic acid, which is found in high concentrations in green leafy vegetables, fruits, orange juice and tomato juice, is important for the prevention of birth defects and pregnancy loss. A high dietary intake of folate coupled with folic acid supplements orally may aid in the prevention of pregnancy complications such as neural tube birth defects.

Folate (*Folic Acid*)				
			$	!
Prevention is the best medicine. If you're pregnant—or looking to be—folic acid is key.	Very strong scientific support.	Easy-to-swallow tablet form is widely available.	Very affordable at under $1/day.	"Likely safe" (NMCD).
18	18	18	18	18
Overall rating: 90%				

Choline, which has a similar biochemical effect to folic acid, also appears to protect against neural tube defects when taken prior to and early in pregnancy.

L-arginine is a semi-essential amino acid needed by the body. Early studies in pregnant women suggest that arginine supplements may improve growth in fetuses that are smaller than average.

Biotin, or vitamin H, is an essential water-soluble B vitamin that has been found to be commonly deficient during pregnancy. Biotin supplementation during pregnancy in not currently standard practice, and prenatal vitamins generally do not contain biotin, but it may be a good idea.

To watch a clip about infertility, scan the QR barcode above into your smart device or enter the following link into your browser: http://bit.ly/QuE9xp

If you're pregnant, you may experience less morning sickness and a greater feeling of well-being by supplementing with vitamin B6. You may also experience less nausea if you take one gram of encapsulated ginger powder each day. And don't forget to prevent dehydration due to morning sickness by refuelling with fluids.

Menopause Support

The hormone replacement therapy component of the Women's Health Initiative study was halted three years early because of small but unacceptable risks of breast cancer, stroke, heart disease and dementia. The results of the WHI are difficult to interpret but have done nothing to lessen interest in alternative remedies for menopausal distress. It seems likely that natural health products can play a supportive role in relieving these symptoms.

Among these alternatives, calcium is the nutrient that has been consistently found to be the most important for attaining peak bone mass and preventing postmenopausal osteoporosis, and adequate vitamin D intake is required for optimal calcium absorption.

Sage, or *Salvia officinalis,* contains compounds with mild estrogenic activity, and in theory at least estrogenic compounds may decrease menopausal symptoms. So far, sage has been tested against menopausal symptoms with promising results.

Some investigators are looking into claims that soy products containing isoflavones may alleviate menopausal symptoms such as hot flashes.

Black cohosh, or *Actaea racemosa*, is popular as an alternative to hormonal therapy in the treatment of menopausal symptoms such as hot flashes, heavy sweating, palpitations, vaginal dryness and mood disturbances.

Black Cohosh (*Actaea racemosa*)				
			$	!
Black cohosh is an excellent alternative for menopausal hormonal symptoms.	Little by way of really compelling science has yet been done.	Easy-to-swallow capsule form is widely available.	Affordable at under $3/day.	"Possibly safe" (NMCD).
18	12	18	16	10
Overall rating: 74%				

MEN'S HEALTH

Protecting and Regulating the Prostate

Pygeum africanum—the African plum tree—is an evergreen of the Rosaceae family that grows in central and southern Africa. Its bark has been used for thousands of years to treat bladder and urination disorders, and in recent studies it has been observed to moderately improve urinary symptoms associated with enlargement of the prostate gland or prostate inflammation. Numerous human studies report that pygeum significantly reduces urinary hesitancy, urinary frequency, the number of times

To watch a clip about prostate support, scan the QR barcode above into your smart device or enter the following link into your browser: http://bit.ly/NsgkG3

patients need to wake up at night to urinate, and pain with urination in men who experience mild-to-moderate symptoms.

Saw palmetto also improves symptoms of benign prostatic hypertrophy such as nighttime urination, urinary flow and overall quality of life.

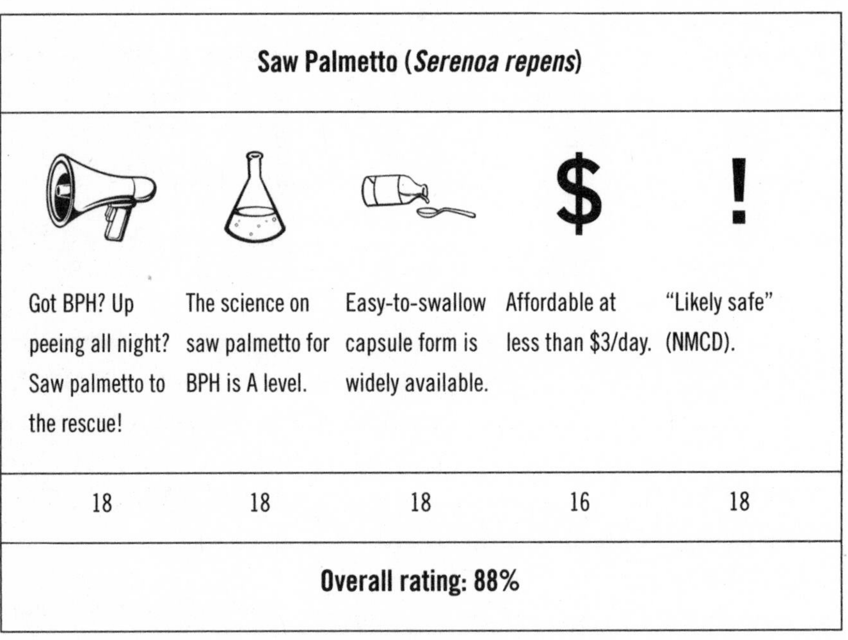

Saw Palmetto (*Serenoa repens*)				
Got BPH? Up peeing all night? Saw palmetto to the rescue!	The science on saw palmetto for BPH is A level.	Easy-to-swallow capsule form is widely available.	Affordable at less than $3/day.	"Likely safe" (NMCD).
18	18	18	16	18
Overall rating: 88%				

Beta-sitosterol is a plant sterol that is present in soybeans, breads, peanuts, fruits, vegetables and the oils of olive, flax seed and tuna. There is some evidence of its efficacy in treating the symptoms of benign prostatic hypertrophy.

Lastly, selenium, a trace mineral found in soil, water and some foods—in particular Brazil nuts—is an essential element in several metabolic pathways. There is some evidence that low selenium levels are associated with an increased risk of prostate cancer. In human studies, initial evidence has suggested that selenium supplementation reduces the risk of developing prostate cancer in men with normal baseline PSA levels and low selenium blood levels.

Men, I hope you don't need me to remind you that the prostate is an important and vulnerable organ. Protect your prostate. Eat more Brazil nuts, get your PSA checked regularly and consider the power found in natural health products.

Erectile Dysfunction

Horny goat weed. Okay, got your attention, right? Believe it or not, that's actually a rough translation of the name for a traditional Chinese medicine, *yin yang huo*, derived from the leaves of the epimedium plant and used in various Chinese medicine herb combinations. The story is that a goatherder found that his male goats became excited after eating from a particular patch of weeds. Needless to say, it's a long way from this story to a reliable application of horny goat weed to male erectile dysfunction, although investigations are under way.

To watch a clip about sexual support, scan the QR barcode above into your smart device or enter the following link into your browser: http://bit.ly/MEC4ic

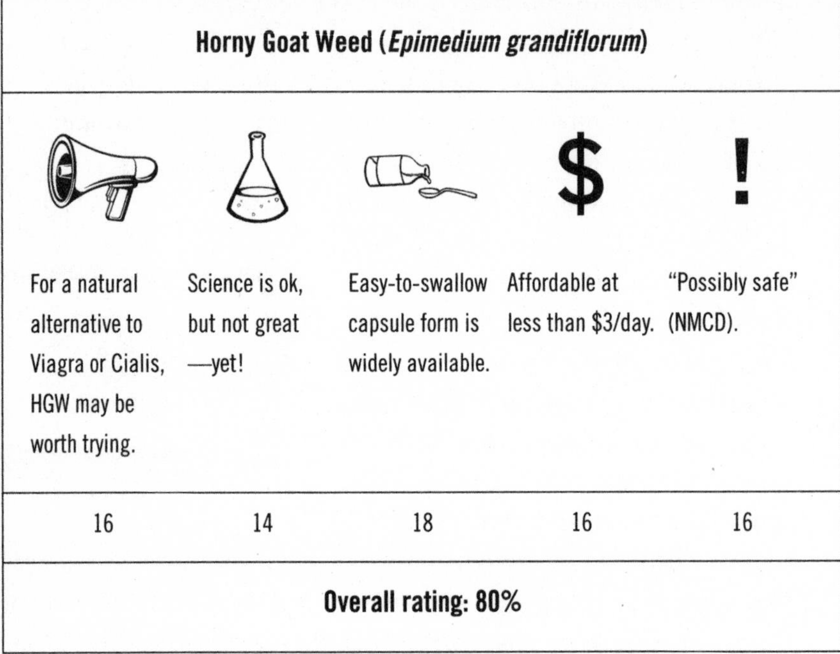

Horny Goat Weed (*Epimedium grandiflorum*)				
For a natural alternative to Viagra or Cialis, HGW may be worth trying.	Science is ok, but not great —yet!	Easy-to-swallow capsule form is widely available.	Affordable at less than $3/day.	"Possibly safe" (NMCD).
16	14	18	16	16
Overall rating: 80%				

Despite the fame and wide adoption of the powerful pharmaceutical sildenafil (trade name Viagra) and related drugs such as Cialis, and the less widely known use of papaverine extract, prostaglandin E1, phentolamine and alprostadil, there are natural alternatives that show real promise. Many are under present investigation.

Asian ginseng may improve libido and the ability to maintain erections.

Yohimbe bark extract contains an active ingredient, yohimbine, that has been proven clinically effective in treating erectile dysfunction by increasing blood flow and dilating blood vessels. However, the amounts of this potent chemical present in the bark extract vary widely and are often unstated.

Arginine is one of the twenty most common amino acids. Taken as a supplement, it can act to dilate blood vessels and has been shown to help men with erectile dysfunction, though with a number of important caveats.

Butea superba is an herb native to Thailand, where it has been used traditionally to increase sexual vigour. In 2003, a randomized double-blind trial examined the effects on erectile dysfuntion of butea in Thai men. About 82 percent of subjects had a noticeable improvement, without any evident toxicities.

To watch a clip about sexual support, scan the QR barcode above into your smart device or enter the following link into your browser: http://bit.ly/MEC4ic

For obvious reasons, there has been an interest in sexual performance enhancers since time immemorial. We can't begin to consider them all here but you might want to read further about ashwagandha herb, catuaba herb, cnidium herb, coleus forskohlii herb, damiana herb, maca extract, passion flower extract, mucuna pruriens extract, muira puama herb, suma herb, rehmannia, rhodiola, shilajit, tribulus and tongkat Ali.

4. WIDE CIRCULATION: SUPPORT FOR OUR HEART AND BLOOD

ANEMIA AND RED BLOOD CELLS

If testing by a qualified health practitioner has determined that you suffer from anemia but have no serious disease, natural health products may be able to boost your red blood cell count to a normal level by replenishing what your body is missing.

Preventing and treating anemia with supplemental iron, vitamin B12 and folic acid is highly effective. Vitamin C may further increase iron absorption.

To watch a clip about red blood cell support, scan the QR barcode above into your smart device or enter the following link into your browser: http://bit.ly/LG5eqU

Interesting new research suggests that the blue-green algae classed as spirulina may help reduce the risk of anemia and increase hemoglobin, especially in the elderly. Also, consuming tofu may help prevent the low red blood cell counts associated with weakness, fatigue and bruising by having a positive effect on iron status, independent of supplemental iron intake.

Blue-Green Algae (*Spirulina*)				
If you're taking iron for anemia, spirulina may enhance the benefits.	So far supported only moderately.	The most available forms—liquid and powder—are not pleasant tasting.	$ Affordable at less than $3/day.	! "Possibly safe" (NMCD).
16	14	14	16	12
Overall rating: 72%				

Blood Sugar: Natural Control

Many studies have shown that alpha lipoic acid may improve blood sugar levels and provide blood glucose support among people with hypoglycemia and type 2 diabetes.

Another excellent natural health product to consider is beta-glucan, a soluble fibre derived from the cell walls of algae, bacteria, fungi, yeast and plants. It is commonly used for its cholesterol-lowering effects but there are several human-trial studies that support the use of beta-glucan for blood sugar control.

A chromium supplement is often recommended to balance blood glucose. And when it comes to herbs, several studies report a blood sugar–lowering effect of American ginseng (*Panax quinquefolium*) in individuals with imbalanced blood sugar.

But the most promising of all is alpha lipoic acid (ALA). ALA is a vitamin-like antioxidant, referred to as the "universal antioxidant" because it is soluble in both fat and water, allowing it to work inside *and* outside your cells. It is one of the best studied supplements for sugar balancing. ALA is manufactured in the body and is found in some foods, particularly liver and yeast. Supplementing with alpha lipoic acid may protect against diabetic complications, such as nerve and kidney damage in type 1 diabetes, and taking alpha lipoic acid may improve insulin

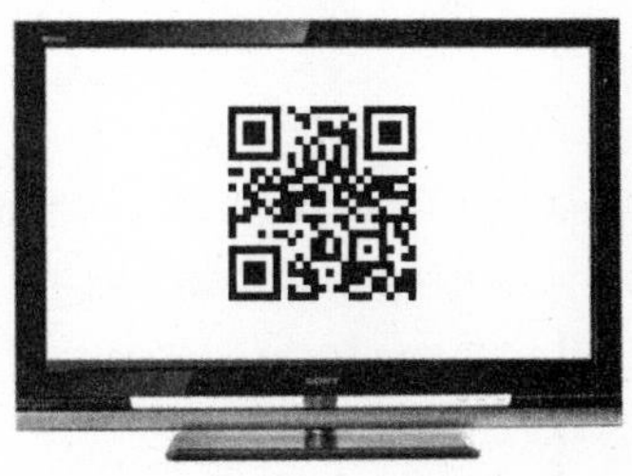

To watch a clip about blood sugar support, scan the QR barcode above into your smart device or enter the following link into your browser: http://bit.ly/QdMF4Y

To watch a clip about alpha lipoic acid, scan the QR barcode above into your smart device or enter the following link into your browser: http://bit.ly/SRcZ2m

sensitivity and help protect against diabetic complications such as nerve damage in type 2.

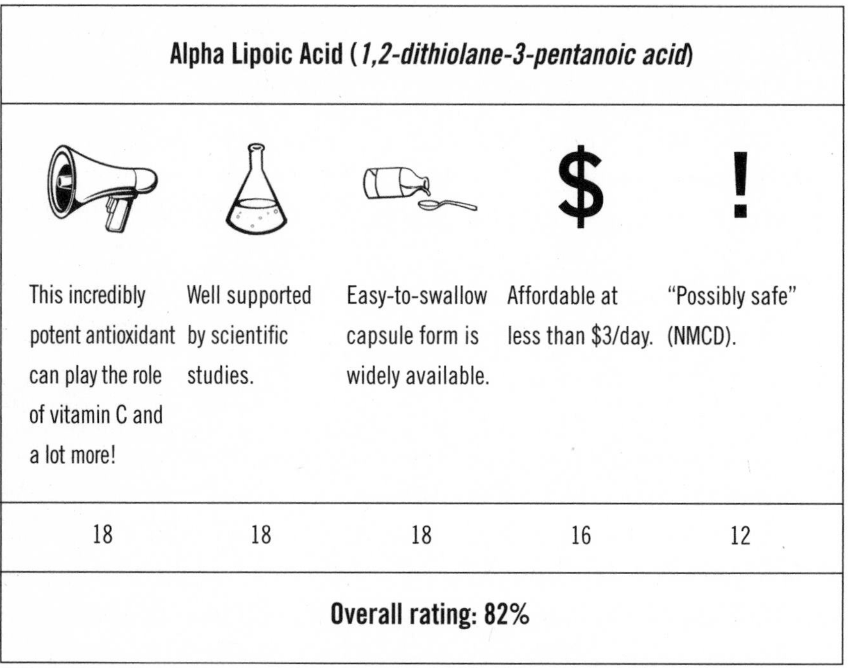

Alpha Lipoic Acid (*1,2-dithiolane-3-pentanoic acid*)				
This incredibly potent antioxidant can play the role of vitamin C and a lot more!	Well supported by scientific studies.	Easy-to-swallow capsule form is widely available.	Affordable at less than $3/day.	"Possibly safe" (NMCD).
18	18	18	16	12
Overall rating: 82%				

Cardiovascular Support

Even if you're in perfect health, you'll want to provide your heart and circulation with every beneficial boost. And if your doctor's investigations—as we discussed in the previous chapter—turn up risk factors (as they often do), these measures may be a matter of life and death.

Beta-sitosterol is found in and synthesized exclusively by plants such as fruits, vegetables, soybeans and peanuts. Beta-sitosterol supplementation has been shown to decrease total serum cholesterol as well as levels of harmful low-density lipoprotein (LDL) cholesterol. It hasn't been proved conclusively but it may be of benefit for people with high levels of blood cholesterol.

Beta-Sitosterol (*22,23-dihydrostigmasterol, 24-ethylcholesterol*)				
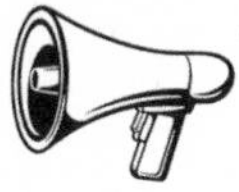	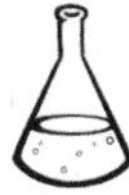	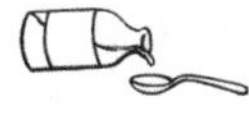	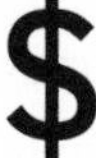	!
Since statin drugs have so many side effects, consider a natural cholesterol-lowering alternative that works.	Beta sitosterol is quite well supported by good studies.	Easy-to-swallow capsule form is widely available	Affordable at less than $3/day.	"Likely safe" (NMCD).
18	16	18	16	16
Overall rating: 84%				

Based on multiple studies, niacin (nicotinic acid) is now a well-accepted and effective natural health treatment for high cholesterol. It has a significantly beneficial effect on levels of high-density cholesterol (HDL, or "good cholesterol"), and on lowering triglycerides with better results than prescription statin drugs. Be sure to use nicotinic acid and not niacinamide, which does not have the same lipid effects.

To watch a clip about heart health and cardiovascular support, scan the QR barcode above into your smart device or enter the following link into your browser: http://bit.ly/NN1UyX

Many studies have also reported reductions in total blood cholesterol and "bad cholesterol" over short periods of time (four to twelve weeks) with the use of garlic. And preliminary human studies suggest that cynarin and artichoke extracts may also have lipid-lowering effects.

Blood Pressure and Natural Health Products

As with conventional drugs, the use of natural substances sometimes controls blood pressure if taken consistently—*but* it doesn't lead to a cure for high blood pressure. Thus, someone whose blood pressure is successfully reduced by weight loss, avoidance of salt and increased intake of fruits and vegetables would need to maintain these changes permanently in order to retain control of blood pressure. That type of intervention is the best and most natural of all. Left untreated, hypertension significantly increases the risk of stroke and heart disease.

We all know that smoking and drinking are particularly injurious for people with hypertension, but the newly identified silent contributor to this problem is stress. We all have to learn ways to relax and de-stress. The combination of obesity, hypertension, smoking, drinking and stress is an invitation for premature suffering and death.

Daily exercise can lower blood pressure significantly. Progressive resistance exercise—for example, weightlifting—also appears to help reduce blood pressure.

There's little doubt that blood pressure can be positively influenced by a diet significantly low in cholesterol and animal fat and high in fresh organic produce, whole grains, legumes and low-fat dairy, with healthy amounts of nuts and seeds. Add ten grams of soy protein or sixteen ounces of soy milk twice daily into your diet to help lower blood pressure. Significantly decrease your salt intake by avoiding the addition of table salt, by limiting your indulgence in salty fast foods and by reading labels in your grocery store to identify low-sodium foods (less than 140 mg per serving).

Various natural health products can be important in helping you lower high blood pressure. One hundred milligrams a day of the powerful antioxidant CoQ10 may have a real impact on your blood pressure after one to several months. Supplements of calcium (800 to 1,500 mg a day) and magnesium (350 to 500 mg a day) may be helpful as well. Try reducing the load on your heart with supplemental garlic: 600 to 900 mg a day of a standardized garlic extract can improve heart and blood vessel health, and also has a mild blood pressure–lowering effect.

To watch a clip about high blood pressure support, scan the QR barcode above into your smart device or enter the following link into your browser: http://bit.ly/P4LW2G

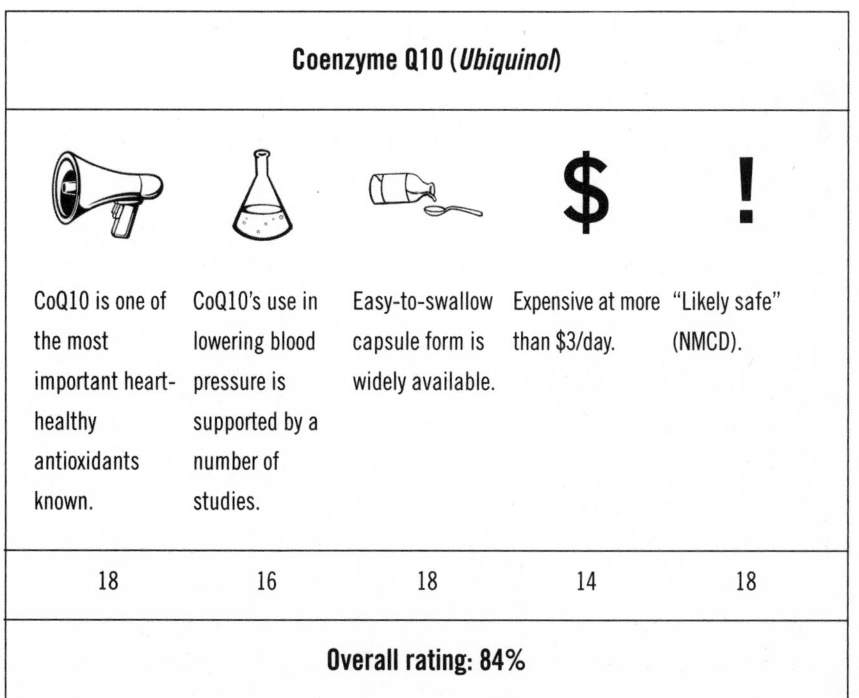

Coenzyme Q10 (*Ubiquinol*)				
CoQ10 is one of the most important heart-healthy antioxidants known.	CoQ10's use in lowering blood pressure is supported by a number of studies.	Easy-to-swallow capsule form is widely available.	Expensive at more than $3/day.	"Likely safe" (NMCD).
18	16	18	14	18
Overall rating: 84%				

Lowering Cholesterol Naturally

Your body obtains cholesterol in two ways: first, by producing the majority of it internally; and second, from dietary sources in the form of animal products such as meats, poultry, fish, eggs, butter, cheese and whole milk. If your levels are high, you're going to want to clean up your diet to help bring them down to normal. Plant foods such as fruits, vegetables and grains do not contain cholesterol. Eat a lot more of those. But much evidence is accumulating to show that eating too many carbohydrates, especially simpler, more refined carbohydrates such as white breads, sugar and pasta may increase levels of triglycerides in the blood, lower the level of high-density lipoprotein (HDL, or "good" cholesterol) and increase low-density lipoprotein (LDL, or "bad" cholesterol). Thus a low-fat diet that includes a higher carbohydrate intake might actually constitute an unhealthy change.

Some of the natural health products we've already discussed can help lower cholesterol. Current evidence tends to support the use of beta-glucan, the soluble fibre derived from the cell walls of algae, bacteria, fungi, yeast and plants, and beta-sitosterol, one of the most common dietary plant sterols synthesized by plants. Many studies have demonstrated its ability to lower total serum cholesterol as well as levels of low-density lipoprotein (LDL—the "bad cholesterol").

To watch a clip about cholesterol support, scan the QR barcode above into your smart device or enter the following link into your browser: http://bit.ly/OUu3zQ

Niacin, or B3, is a well-accepted treatment for high cholesterol, and there is strong scientific evidence from human trials that omega-3 fatty acids from fish or fish oil supplements (EPA and DHA) significantly reduce blood triglyceride levels. Also psyllium, which is derived from the husks of the seeds of *Plantago ovata,* contains a high level of soluble dietary fibre, and is well studied as a cholesterol-lowering agent. Lastly, since 1970, human studies have reported that red yeast rice extract lowers blood levels of total cholesterol, low-density lipoprotein/LDL and triglycerides. In fact, the statin drugs (e.g., Lipitor and Crestor) are all derived from red yeast rice. It is now difficult to find red yeast rice on the market that contains the active "statin" ingredient.

5. COMPOS MENTIS: SUPPORT FOR OUR NERVOUS SYSTEM

Modern neuroscience has confirmed what seems like common sense: keeping the brain active increases its vitality and provides positive support for the entire nervous system. Reading, learning a new language, doing crossword puzzles, remaining socially and physically active, having fun—in fact, almost anything new and stimulating counts as increased brain activity.

I find that many people rarely think of alternative medicine when they think about mental health. Conventional psychopharmacology has brought us some powerful weapons that help allay the symptoms of serious mental illness such as schizophrenia, but the scientific investigation of alternative therapies and remedies is ongoing and of great interest to researchers. Meanwhile, mental health means much more than staying out of an institution. It means living our inner lives as fully as possible. The aches and pains of our psychic selves are just as real as those of our physical bodies and it's here that a multitude of alternative approaches can make a real contribution.

GENERAL SUPPORT FOR THE NERVOUS SYSTEM

Good, ongoing clinical research suggests that DHA is only the best researched of a raft of nutrients and botanicals—alpha

To watch a clip about nervous system support, scan the QR barcode above into your smart device or enter the following link into your browser: http://bit.ly/SQSIQ6

lipoic acid, huperzine A, vinpocetine, astaxanthin, bacopa, citicoline and others—that have neuroprotective effects and support mental energy, focus, vigilance and memory.

Astaxanthin, found in high concentrations in salmon, in certain other fish and in fruit like mangoes, blueberries and cranberries, is a powerful antioxidant classed as a natural health product that may help prevent nerve degeneration.

INSOMNIA

We go to bed but can't fall asleep. We wake up in the middle of the night and can't get back to sleep. Insomnia, the prolonged inability to get adequate sleep, can be a temporary, occasional or chronic problem, but we know it has been found to reduce memory and focus, and can impair the general functioning of our nervous system.

Our first strategy for dealing with insomnia is to create a restful place to sleep. Remove or block noise, light and other distractions, and make sure your mattress is comfortable. We call these steps "sleep hygiene." Ideal sleep hygiene also includes room temperature, which should be set between 65 and 72 degrees Fahrenheit.

Next comes what *not* to take. Cut down on coffee and on drinks, foods and medicine that contain caffeine, ephedra, or pseudoephedrine and other stimulants. Work with your doctor to find alternatives if you take medication with any of these ingredients.

You can't sleep if you're not relaxed and there is an abundance of relaxation tapes and other self-help tools to combat insomnia. You may also consider seeing a counsellor who specializes in cognitive behavioural therapy or who is experienced in treating this disorder.

Valerian is an herb native to Europe and Asia but it now grows almost everywhere. The name suggests the Latin word "valere"—healthy or strong—and it's the root of the valerian plant that seems to contain the active constituents. Valerian has been used to treat insomnia and anxiety for a very long time and some human studies seem to suggest that it improves the quality of sleep, especially when used on an ongoing basis by poor sleepers. I wouldn't regard the research to date as conclusive, but I do recommend that you try 300 to 600 mg of a concentrated root extract thirty minutes before bedtime, with or without other relaxing herbs, such as lemon balm and passion flower, and try this over an extended period, say, three weeks, to see whether you fall asleep more readily and enjoy deeper sleep quality.

To watch a clip about sleep support, scan the QR barcode above into your smart device or enter the following link into your browser: http://bit.ly/M6ocNH

Valerian (*Valeriana officinalis L.*)				
			$	!
Valerian is the most popular herb used for relaxation, anxiety and depression.	Mediocre science but I anticipate more robust investigation in the near future.	Easy-to-swallow capsule and widely available.	Affordable at about $2/day.	"Likely safe" (NMCD).
18	14	18	16	18
Overall rating: 86%				

To watch a clip about pumpkin seed extract for sleep, scan the QR barcode above into your smart device or enter the following link into your browser: http://bit.ly/M6zt01

Melatonin is a hormone produced in the brain by the pineal gland from the amino acid tryptophan—yes, that's the same tryptophan that is famously present in turkey meat. The natural release of melatonin is stimulated by darkness and suppressed by light and blood melatonin levels are highest at bedtime. All this suggests that melatonin is involved in circadian rhythm and the regulation of the body's functions. That's why synthetic melatonin supplements have been widely studied for their effects on sleep and a variety of related disorders. The studies have not been absolutely rigorous but the results persuade me that, if you suffer from insomnia, you should try about 1 mg of melatonin per 25 pounds of body weight. Some of my patients take tryptophan—the precursor to melatonin—prior to bedtime and find it very helpful. Considering the soporific effects of a big turkey dinner at Thanksgiving, they may be right. And speaking of Thanksgiving, pumpkin seed extract—commercially available as a pulverized pumpkin seed powder—is a wonderful natural health product that seems to act as a timed-release mechanism of tryptophan to induce healthy and deep sleep through the night.

Melatonin (*N-acetyl-5-methoxytryptamine*)				
			$	!
Melatonin is an effective sleep aid and when taken properly cures jet lag.	Numerous studies suggest the efficacy of melatonin.	Easy to take in strips, liquid and capsule form and widely available.	Affordable at less than $2/day.	"Likely safe" (NMCD).
18	17	18	16	18
Overall rating: 87%				

STRESS AND ANXIETY

Natural therapies and natural health products can play a role in helping to relieve mild to moderate anxiety.

The first step is often to reduce exposure to stressful situations—without engaging in extreme avoidance behaviours that can themselves be disabling. A person who attempted to deal with a phobia of automobiles by never getting in a car again might make a minuscule contribution to improving the environment but would most certainly encumber and limit his or her life in the twenty-first century. That's why professionals try to deal with anxiety disorders by addressing the problem's roots within the individual personality. Therapeutic approaches based on meditation, counselling or group therapy have all proved to be helpful if properly administered. A form of counselling known as cognitive-behavioural therapy (CBT) has been shown to work well in managing the symptoms of panic disorder, an especially unpleasant form of acute anxiety.

To watch a clip about stress and anxiety support, scan the QR barcode above into your smart device or enter the following link into your browser: http://bit.ly/NHdMkw

There is a wide range of natural health products that have been used to address anxiety. A formidable trio is supplemental B complex, magnesium and 5-HTP (5-hydroxytryptophan). The third of these is the precursor of the neurotransmitter serotonin and is obtained commercially from the seeds of the plant *Griffonia simplicifolia*. Evidence suggests that the three together help battle stress and relieve anxiety.

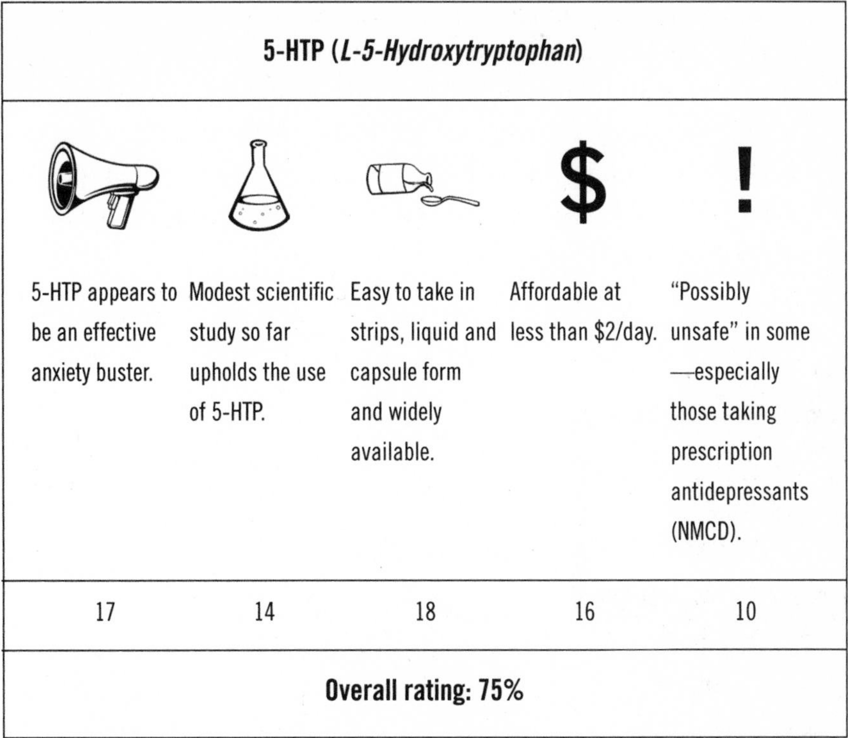

5-HTP (*L-5-Hydroxytryptophan*)				
5-HTP appears to be an effective anxiety buster.	Modest scientific study so far upholds the use of 5-HTP.	Easy to take in strips, liquid and capsule form and widely available.	Affordable at less than $2/day.	"Possibly unsafe" in some —especially those taking prescription antidepressants (NMCD).
17	14	18	16	10
Overall rating: 75%				

Finally, we certainly should not ignore chamomile tea at bedtime. Chamomile has been used medicinally for thousands of years, often specifically for anxiety and insomnia, and modern studies appear to support its traditional uses.

Recent research has also demonstrated that fish oil—which as we've seen has proven cardiac benefits—significantly outperforms placebos in improving anxiety levels for substance abusers.

Inositol, a modified form of vitamin B3, has been used to help reduce the misery of panic attacks.

In combination, passion flower extract and valerian have been shown to reduce symptoms in people suffering from anxiety. A similar effect has been reported regarding St. John's wort.

American skullcap and the hop plant used to flavour beer are part of a group of traditional "nerve tonic" (or nervine) herbs, as is bacopa, the herb used in Ayurvedic medicine.

A recent study suggests that the roots of the *Rhodiola rosea* plant, which grows in the frigid mountain regions of Europe, North America and Asia, may significantly improve generalized anxiety disorder symptoms.

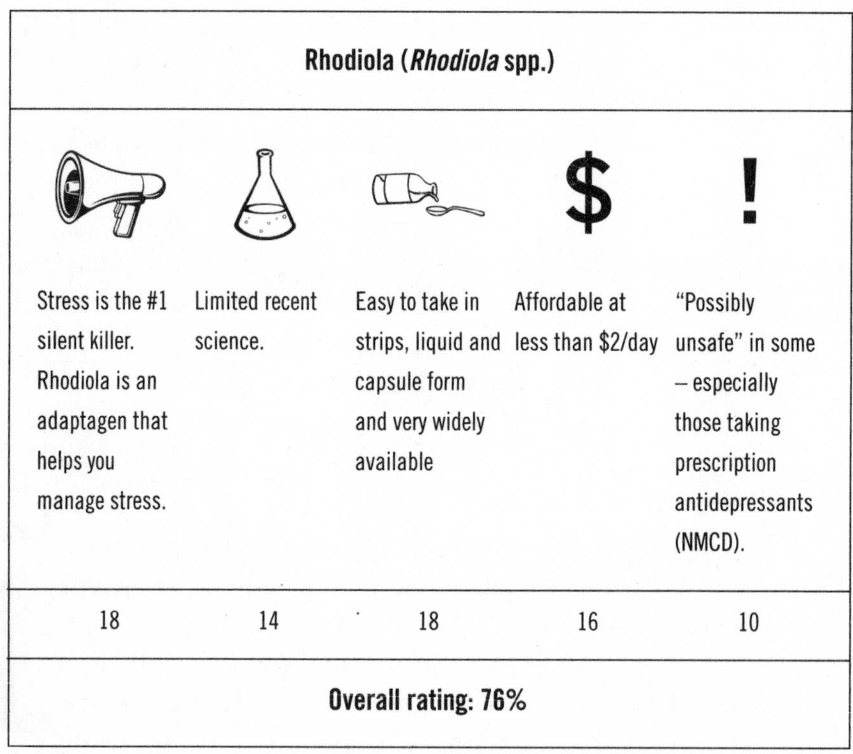

Rhodiola (*Rhodiola* spp.)				
			$	!
Stress is the #1 silent killer. Rhodiola is an adaptagen that helps you manage stress.	Limited recent science.	Easy to take in strips, liquid and capsule form and very widely available	Affordable at less than $2/day	"Possibly unsafe" in some – especially those taking prescription antidepressants (NMCD).
18	14	18	16	10
Overall rating: 76%				

Homeopathic remedies such as the aconite plant, gelsemium and argentum nitricum are considered powerful agents for dealing with anxiety and stress-related symptoms. There are no toxicity issues with these remedies but they require experienced matching of the remedy to the specific symptom in order to work.

MEMORY AIDS

It is generally accepted that aging and memory loss go together, but it's also known that there are ways of keeping our aging brains sharp. Staying active both mentally and physically can help prevent memory loss. Most of us think gingko when we think of an herb with memory-boosting effects. However, where gingko shows some effectiveness in the treatment of dementia (multi-infarct and Alzheimer's type), it appears to have only weak potency in improving the memory of healthy patients. New research, however, suggests that the herb bacopa might offer additional memory benefits. One study, published in the *Journal of Alternative and Complementary Medicine*, included 98 healthy people over 55 years old. They were randomly assigned to receive either 300 mg of *Bacopa monnieri* extract per day or placebo for twelve weeks. Memory and learning tests done at the beginning and end of the trial included tasks such as remembering lists of words, re-creating complicated geometric shapes from memory, and following letter and number patterns. Participants also answered questions about recent memory changes. The authors of the study concluded that bacopa significantly improves memory acquisition and retention in older Australians. This study was well designed and executed but of course an improvement on one test does not prove decisively that bacopa improves memory acquisition and retention. Like most studies it had some limitations and bears repeating and refinement.

The take-away for us is that natural and traditional health products often stand up to scientific scrutiny and that this work has barely begun. Every one of us can benefit from greater awareness of the latest developments.

Bacopa (*Bacopa monnieri*)				
Bacopa may be the answer for a sharper memory.	Supported by some good studies.	Easy-to-swallow capsule and widely available.	Affordable at less than $2/day.	"Possibly safe" (NMCD).
16	16	18	16	12
Overall rating: 78%				

Vinpocetine is an extract of the periwinkle plant that has also been shown to significantly increase memory and focus. We'll look at it more closely when we discuss the drastic memory loss associated with dementia.

DEMENTIA

In 1948, a group of American researchers began a study of heart disease that followed 5,209 adults living in the town of Framingham, Massachusetts. That now-famous study has given us much of what we know about the causes of heart disease. Other Framingham-based research has joined the great heart study, and in 2006 follow-up work demonstrated that an omega-3 fatty acid called DHA decreases the risk of developing all-cause dementia by 47 percent.

This is just a staggering number but maybe it's not surprising. I call DHA omega-3 "brain juice" because it makes up 40 to 60 percent of our brain. It's the motor oil of our mental engine that can stave off the "brain breakdown" that seems to come with modern nutritional habits and stress. By the way, DHA itself is also vital to pregnant and nursing moms because it's important for the development of the baby's brain and eye health and may actually raise the newborn's IQ.

So based on these studies and others continuing, I'm recommending 180 mg of DHA a day—that's two teaspoons—a pretty painless alternative to the tragedy of depression and dementia.

Also, a supplement known as vinpocetine, which is derived from the periwinkle plant, has proven clinical benefit for patients with central nervous system disorders and psychosyndromes, such as dementia. It is best known for its ability to protect the nerves responsible for thought. It has been used to maintain and improve brain health and cognition and shown to cause relaxation of smooth muscle, thereby improving blood flow, oxygen and nutrients in the brain, which in turn improve cerebral efficiency.

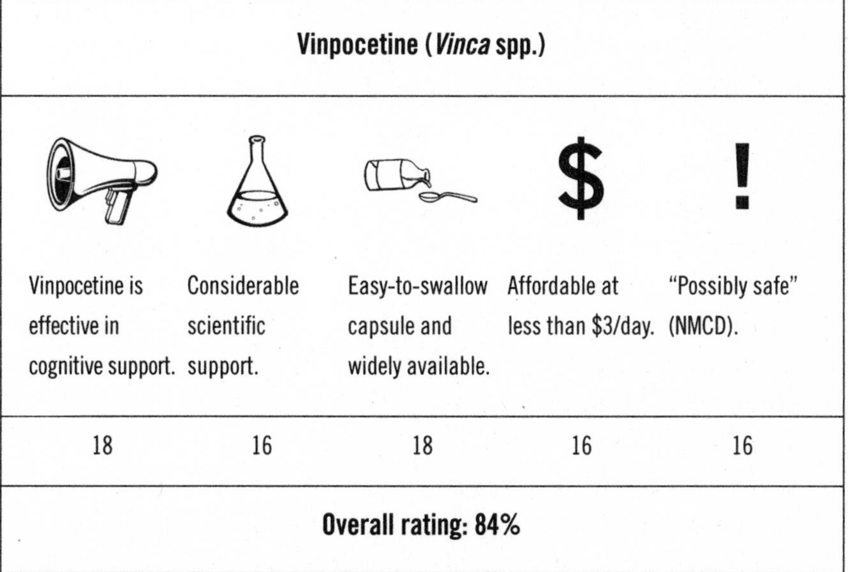

Vinpocetine (*Vinca* spp.)				
			$	!
Vinpocetine is effective in cognitive support.	Considerable scientific support.	Easy-to-swallow capsule and widely available.	Affordable at less than $3/day.	"Possibly safe" (NMCD).
18	16	18	16	16
Overall rating: 84%				

To watch a clip about herbal healers including vinpocetine, scan the QR barcode above into your smart device or enter the following link into your browser: http://bit.ly/MESBT4

ELECTROMAGMETIC FREQUENCY RADIATION: A CAUTION

Several studies have suggested that using a cellphone frequently over ten years or more can cause, or increase the risk of, brain cancer, salivary gland tumours, Alzheimer's disease and behaviour problems. But not all cellphones are created equal: some brands and models emit more electromagnetic frequency radiation (or EMF) than others and a device can have different radiation levels when paired with different service providers. The key factors seem to be the level of radiation emitted, for how long, and from what distance to your body, especially your head. I personally recommend that you investigate the phone you're presently using, switch to a safer phone if you can identify one, limit exposure by using a headset and holding the phone away from your head when talking, and toting your cell in a purse instead of your pocket. And score one for the teens: texting emits far less EMF than talking.

6. DEALING WITH PAIN: NATURAL RELIEF FOR CHRONIC CONDITIONS

In the previous chapter we talked about the paradox of pain: the indispensable warning mechanism that is humankind's greatest affliction, ultimately trumping death as our worst fear. It's small wonder that remedies for pain have long figured so centrally in medicine and small wonder too that many of these remedies, addressing as they do a mechanism so profound, have terrible effects of their own.

From a pharmacological point of view (the mechanism of action on the body), the term "analgesic" is used to define ingredients that give us the feeling that pain is reduced. In reality, an analgesic blocks or stops the signal of pain to the brain, which would normally interpret this signal to tell us that it hurts. Even modern pharmaceuticals such as aspirin, acetaminophen and ibuprofen carry serious potential risk. Compared to many other analgesics, acetaminophen (Tylenol) has had a relatively good safety profile, its most common side effect being nausea, but recent studies confirm that even low dosages may cause liver toxicity, especially when taken chronically. The more effective narcotic analgesics carry notorious risks of toxicity and addiction. That's why traditional medicine and modern natural medicine have constantly sought alternatives such as acupuncture, electrical stimulation and nerve blocking.

When it comes to serious pain, natural medicine may not pack the hefty punch that the intense prescription analgesics do. However, natural medications, like some of the non-medicinal pain-relieving procedures that are beyond the scope of this book, can effectively reduce the dosages of the pharmaceutical drug of choice to avoid undesirable side effects or simply to increase the therapeutic effectiveness. For example, adding stinging nettle to non-steroidal anti-inflammatory (NSAID) therapy such as ibuprofen may increase anti-inflammatory activity and avoid having to raise the dosage level of the NSAID. Since pain may prevent you from falling asleep or from having a restful sleep, you may also want to consider some of the sleep aids we've discussed. When it comes to pain associated with fibromyalgia in particular, numerous studies have shown that restful sleep is a key element to recovery.

Bromelain is a sulphur-containing digestive enzyme that is extracted from the stem and the fruit of the pineapple plant. Its

To watch a clip about pain support, scan the QR barcode above into your smart device or enter the following link into your browser: http://bit.ly/PMxgmm

use as an anti-inflammatory agent and its application to sinusitis has been substantiated by clinical evidence and there is some evidence to support its effectiveness for arthritis and muscle pain.

Three species of comfrey (*Symphytum spp.*) appear to be medicinally significant and these have been traditionally used topically for inflammation, pain and wound healing. Clinical trials investigating the topical application of comfrey-containing creams have found significant reductions in inflammation and pain associated with sprains and muscle injuries.

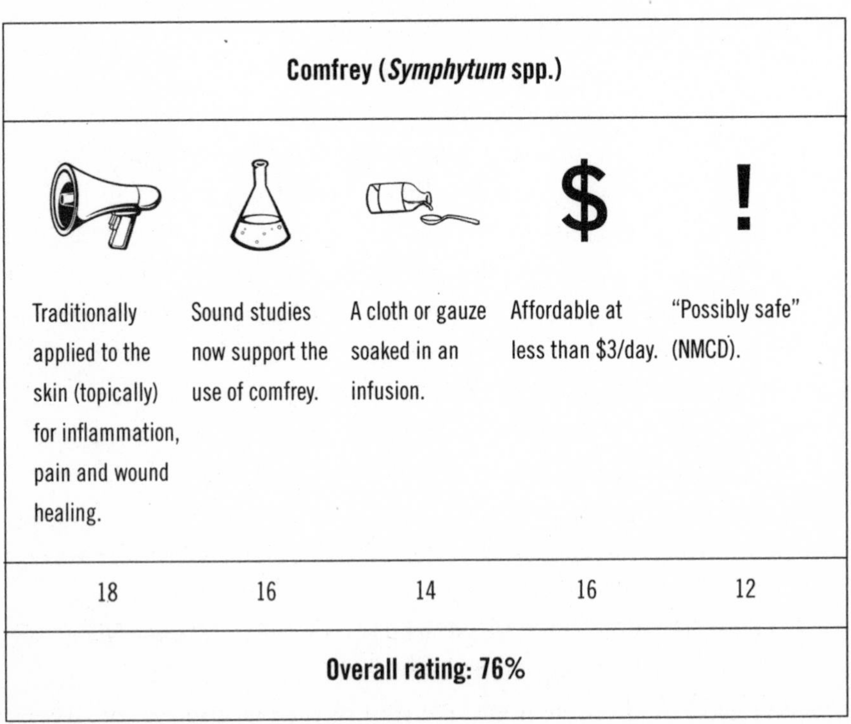

Comfrey (*Symphytum* spp.)				
Traditionally applied to the skin (topically) for inflammation, pain and wound healing.	Sound studies now support the use of comfrey.	A cloth or gauze soaked in an infusion.	Affordable at less than $3/day.	"Possibly safe" (NMCD).
18	16	14	16	12
Overall rating: 76%				

Extract from devil's claw *(Harpagophytum procumbens)*, which originates in the Kalahari and savannah desert regions of southern and southeastern Africa, has been convincingly demonstrated to be effective in the treatment of low back pain and muscular pain. Combining devil's claw with California poppy is especially powerful as a pain relief regimen that is non-addictive by comparison with most conventional drug approaches that offer the same effectiveness.

To watch a clip that considers some complementary alternative medicine to common prescriptions (including California poppy), scan the QR barcode above into your smart device or enter the following link into your browser: http://bit.ly/NRCkpt

Devil's Claw (*Harpagophytum procumbens*)				
Devil's claw is a natural alternative to ulcer-promoting anti-inflammatory drugs.	Supported by sound studies.	Easy-to-swallow capsule and widely available.	Affordable at less than $2/day.	"Possibly safe" (NMCD).
18	16	18	16	12
Overall rating: 80%				

To watch a clip about devil's claw, scan the QR barcode above into your smart device or enter the following link into your browser: http://bit.ly/MjYhNQ

And no discussion of pain could be complete without mentioning toothache. The essential oil of cloves is commonly used as a dental pain reliever and in fact is the most effective natural health product known for this application. Early studies have found that a homemade clove gel may be as effective as benzocaine topically. You just apply it directly to the affected site and get yourself to the dentist. Clove oil combined with zinc oxide paste may also be effective for dry socket, a temporary but painful complication that sometimes happens after a tooth is removed.

ARTHRITIS SUPPORT

Although there is currently no cure for osteoarthritis or rheumatoid arthritis, natural health products can help reduce tissue degeneration, swelling and pain and help people suffering from these diseases to remain active.

If you have arthritis, eat more avocado and fish. The regular intake of fish and fish oil supplements has shown promising results in the control of inflammation in the joints. This is especially true for fish oils high in EPA, the omega-3 with strong anti-inflammatory action.

A lot of evidence also supports the use of oral glucosamine and chondroitin. Glucosamine is a natural compound that is found in healthy cartilage and strong evidence based on human trials supports its use in the treatment of mild-to-moderate knee osteoarthritis.

Preliminary evidence suggests that gamma linolenic acid (or GLA) from borage seed oil may have anti-inflammatory effects that may make it beneficial in treating rheumatoid arthritis.

Devil's claw is a safe and beneficial herb for the short-term treatment of pain related to degenerative joint disease or osteoarthritis and may be as effective as non-steroidal anti-inflammatory drugs such as ibuprofen but without the side effects including gastric ulcers.

And again, some evidence supports the possible effectiveness of bromelain for arthritic pain.

To watch a clip about arthritis support, scan the QR barcode above into your smart device or enter the following link into your browser: http://bit.ly/PDJxts

FIBROMYALGIA SUPPORT

Various medications, behavioural interventions, support groups, patient education and exercise have been found effective in reducing fibromyalgia symptoms. In mild cases, a reduction in stress and certain lifestyle changes may be enough to manage the disease. These changes may include participation in counselling, regular exercise, physical therapy, healthy sleep habits and stress reduction.

Natural health products can play a significant role in treatment of fibromyalgia by providing relief of symptoms. Of note is hydroxy-tryptophan (5-HTP), the precursor of the neurotransmitter serotonin that is obtained commercially from the seeds of the griffonia plant. Some research has been conducted to evaluate the use of 5-HTP for fibromyalgia, and early evidence suggests that it may reduce the number of tender points, anxiety and intensity of pain, and may improve sleep, fatigue and morning stiffness.

To watch a clip about fibromyalgia support, scan the QR barcode above into your smart device or enter the following link into your browser: http://bit.ly/MEpa3D

A randomized controlled trial and one case series indicate that chlorella—a green algae supplement—may also reduce the tenderness associated with fibromyalgia's tender points.

Lastly, although not yet studied in fibromyalgia, California poppy may be of real benefit since it has analgesic properties, sleep-inducing properties, and is not addictive.

7. AS TIME GOES BY: GETTING AND STAYING HEALTHY AS WE AGE

REINING IN THE FREE RASCALS

In the previous chapter, I said a little about some of the profound mechanisms that underlie aging. In particular I explained how the oxygen molecules called "free radicals" cause such widespread damage to our bodies.

Some foods and herbals are identified as "antioxidants" because they have the ability to neutralize the free radical molecules. It's a reasonable assumption therefore that antioxidants are generally good for us and supplementation with such antioxidants as resveratrol—found in the skin of the red grape—is showing promise as an anti-aging agent.

In my previous book, *The Antioxidant Prescription*, I look in detail at the issue of free radicals and how to limit their damage.

TELOMERES: THE LONG AND THE SHORT AND THE SMALL

We earlier discussed the telomere mechanism. It's complex and not fully understood, but it now seems as though our old friends the omega-3 fatty acids may slow the rate of shortening of telomere length and so help prevent age-related muscle loss, among other things.

A New York–based company, T.A. Sciences, manufactures a

supplement in pill form that has been lab tested and shown to stop telomeres from shortening. Their product, TA-65, comes from extracts of the herb astragalus, which has been used over the last thousand years for many medicinal purposes including allergic rhinitis, the common cold, hepatitis and even cancer. TA-65 is produced at very low levels in the astragalus plant, but T.A. Sciences purifies and concentrates the substance, which is thought to "turn on" the enzyme telomerase (hTERT) that acts to maintain or lengthen telomeres and therefore slow down aging.

To watch a clip about anti-aging support, scan the QR barcode above into your smart device or enter the following link into your browser: http://bit.ly/QdLqTw

TRADITIONAL PRACTICES

Through the ages, cultures have developed practices intended to slow the aging process. Ashwagandha has been used in Indian Ayurvedic medicine for many centuries as an aid in slowing aging, promoting physical and mental health and improving resistance to disease. Yoga also originated as meditation-with-movement in India. Tai chi, the system of movements and positions believed to have developed in twelfth-century China, aims to address the body and mind as an interconnected system. Tai chi is traditionally believed to have mental and physical health benefits to improve posture, balance, flexibility and strength and may slow aging by improving overall physical functioning and sense of well-being. These systems have survived for centuries and deserve our respect and attention, so if you are interested, it's worth looking at the literature that discusses these various practices.

BUILDING BONES

Somehow, bones and aging are often linked in common parlance. Maybe it's because our bony skeletons are emblems of death or maybe it's because some of the most common and painful aspects of aging—aching joints and limbs—are associated with our bones. Yet the fact is that with favourable genetics, proper nourishment, a healthy lifestyle and weight-bearing exercise, healthy bones *do* last a lifetime.

Calcium and phosphorus are obviously essential for healthy bone formation, since the bony part of bone is largely a complex calcium phosphate. But magnesium and trace minerals are also important. These include the often forgotten boron, strontium, zinc and manganese. Vitamins D and K are also key, and in fact vitamin D3, or cholecalciferol, is the single most important factor in the absorption of calcium. Although humans are fully capable of making vitamin D, this process is dependent upon adequate exposure to the UVB rays of the sun, not so easy for people who are often confined indoors because of climate or their health. Vitamin K knits the bones together, regulating calcium in bone and keeping it out of soft tissue. (The last thing we'd want would be to have stiff arteries.)

To watch a clip about building stronger bones and bone support, scan the QR barcode above into your smart device or enter the following link into your browser: http://bit.ly/P3UaYZ

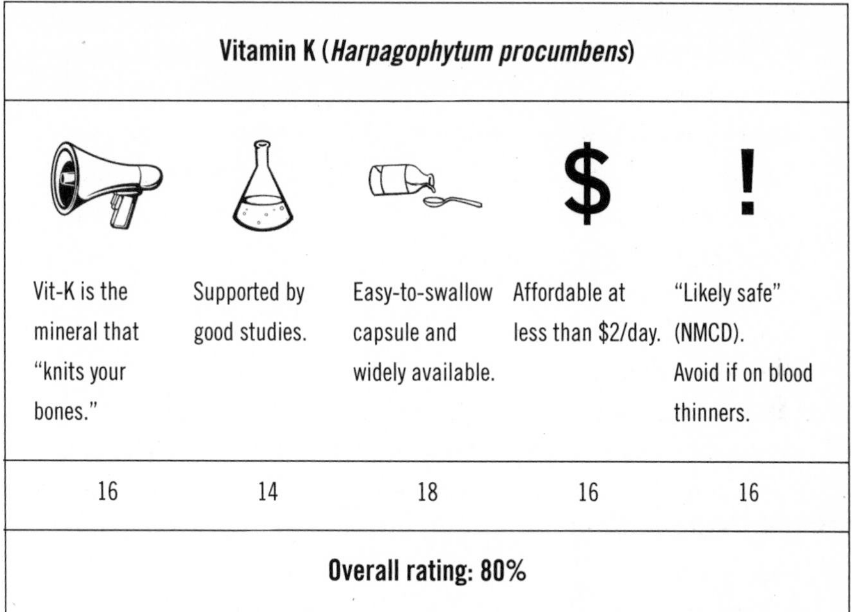

Vitamin K (*Harpagophytum procumbens*)				
Vit-K is the mineral that "knits your bones."	Supported by good studies.	Easy-to-swallow capsule and widely available.	Affordable at less than $2/day.	"Likely safe" (NMCD). Avoid if on blood thinners.
16	14	18	16	16
Overall rating: 80%				

ENERGY AND STAMINA

In the last chapter we talked about noradrenalin, the "happy hormone," and the importance of its proper functioning in the brain if we want to keep that energized feeling. Running your brain with low noradrenalin is akin to running your car with a failing battery. Sooner or later, it just won't start. But a class of natural health products called "adaptogens" may be an effective solution. Adaptogens regulate stress resistance and increase performance, energy and endurance. Extracts of the roots of the *Rhodiola rosea* plant, which we met earlier when we looked at remedies for anxiety, is an excellent example of an adaptogen that is believed to normalize functioning and stimulate healing of cells. It has been used to prevent fatigue and enhance physical and mental performance.

Just as important as raising the levels of the "happy hormone" is lowering chronically high levels of cortisol, adrenaline and other stress hormones. Since these are naturally present at higher levels in the morning, exercising at the start of the day can help you metabolize them more quickly. Don't have more than one coffee. Cut out high glycemic index foods that spike blood sugar and cause mid-morning crashes that zap noradrenalin and energy. For the same reason, consider ten minutes of deep breathing or meditation using biofeedback concepts.

Sleep—especially so-called deep phase-four sleep—recharges your adrenal glands. This sort of recharge is akin to trickle-charging a battery. On the other hand, "boosting" with caffeine and sugar is like jump charging. They have the effect of eventually burning out your energy-replenishment system. You'll find it increasingly difficult to keep a charge and you'll often crave compensatory boosts: sedatives at night such as alcohol, prescription drugs or more food. If you do require supplemental sleep aids, remember the natural products such as melatonin, grifonia seed and pumpkin seed powder that we looked at earlier.

A very well known natural energy booster is ginseng. Ginseng's actions in the body are thought to be due to a complex interplay of constituents. Traditionally it is taken as an energy booster and tonic. There is scientific evidence regarding the effect of ginseng on exercise capacity, cognitive performance and well-being. The primary ingredient is the ginsenoside, which is believed to counter the effects of stress and enhance intellectual and physical performance.

To watch a clip about energy and stamina support, scan the QR barcode above into your smart device or enter the following link into your browser: http://bit.ly/P4AfJh

Although there are no human clinical trials, adaptogenic herbs such as Asian ginseng may be useful for people with chronic fatigue syndrome, it is thought to have an immuno-modulating effect and thereby help support the normal function of the person with chronic fatigue feel more energy.

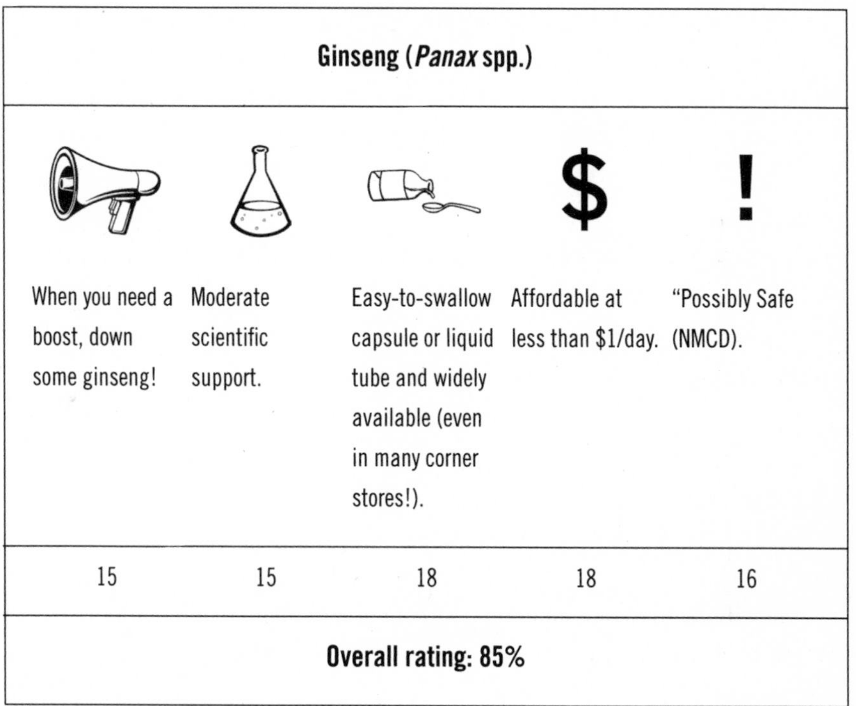

Ginseng (*Panax* spp.)				
When you need a boost, down some ginseng!	Moderate scientific support.	Easy-to-swallow capsule or liquid tube and widely available (even in many corner stores!).	Affordable at less than $1/day.	"Possibly Safe (NMCD).
15	15	18	18	16
Overall rating: 85%				

HORMONAL SUPPORT

In the previous chapter, we looked at tests for blood, urine and salivary hormone markers. If the results suggest reason for concern, what can we do?

The modern farming industry is under pressure to produce animals and vegetation destined for consumption at a predetermined weight and size, in the shortest time and at the lowest possible cost. This demand has led to the use of growth-promotion techniques, including antibiotics in feed, as well as naturally occurring and man-made steroid hormones administered during the growth phase. Obviously the ingestion of random hormones puts your hormonal balance at risk. That's why conscientious health practitioners recommend purchasing and consuming organic foods as much as possible.

Men and women have quite different hormone balances in their bodies. For women, a natural health product that can ensure the body's hormones remain in balance is Vitex, commonly called chasteberry, whose benefits stem from its actions upon the pituitary gland and specifically on the production of the luteinizing hormone. This hormone indirectly increases progesterone production and helps regulate the menstrual cycle. Vitex also keeps prolactin secretion in check, which may benefit some infertile women as well as those with breast tenderness associated with premenstrual syndrome.

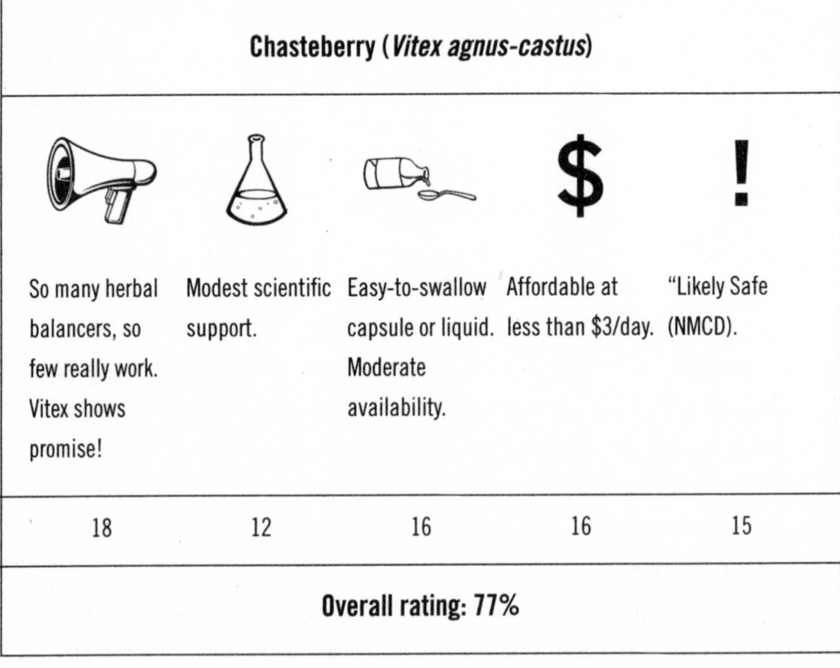

Chasteberry (*Vitex agnus-castus*)				
			$	!
So many herbal balancers, so few really work. Vitex shows promise!	Modest scientific support.	Easy-to-swallow capsule or liquid. Moderate availability.	Affordable at less than $3/day.	"Likely Safe (NMCD).
18	12	16	16	15
Overall rating: 77%				

For men, one of the more popular hormonal balancers is maca root. Maca, found wild in Peru, Bolivia, Paraguay and Argentina, has been cultivated as a root crop for at least two thousand years. Traditionally it has been used to relieve stress, as an aphrodisiac and for fertility enhancement, but more recently, maca products have gained considerable popularity, with claims that they can boost energy, balance hormones and enhance sexual performance. I have some doubts about these claims, but maca root does have some mediocre science to support claims that it's an aphrodisiac, that it helps with hormone regulation and that it improves spermatogenesis (sperm health) in men.

THE BATTLE AGAINST INFLAMMATION

If you have an inflammatory disorder such as inflammatory bowel disease, talk with your doctor, nutritionist or other health-care professional about which specific nutrients and foods may support and optimize your health.

One of the most important dietary discoveries in recent times is the fact that one of the many functions of prostaglandins—which are derived from fats—is to either decrease or increase inflammation, depending on which kind of fat they're derived from. We know—or we should know by now—that the "bad" fats include the polyunsaturates and transfatty acids. The "good" fats are the omega-3 fatty acids found in foods such as cold-water fish and nuts, and they have a wide range of important health benefits. A recent study reported in the *American Journal of Clinical Nutrition* found that nuts may help lower by more than 30 percent a person's risk of dying from inflammation-based diseases such as inflammatory bowel disease, asthma and rheumatoid arthritis. (And by the way, watch out when you see that magic word "omega." The typical North American diet includes more omega-6 than omega-3 fatty acids, yet it's omega-3 that health experts recommend we need more of for optimal health. In fact, too much omega-6 can actually contribute to chronic inflammation.

Fish and nuts are not the only foods to combat inflammation. Many foods high in vitamins A, C and E play a valuable role. Fruits including blackberries, strawberries, raspberries, kiwi, peaches, mangoes, cantaloupe and apples have been shown to be anti-inflammatory. A new study has found that blood antioxidant levels were significantly higher and inflammatory levels significantly lower after the ingestion of the pomegranate extract. Many vegetables including carrots, squash, sweet potato, spinach, kale, collard greens, broccoli, cabbage and Brussels sprouts have anti-inflammatory effects, as do grains including lentils, chickpeas, brown rice, wheat germ and non-instant oatmeal.

I find it interesting that some of our more exotic spices are notably anti-inflammatory. Turmeric, with its active phytonutrient curcumin, has significant anti-inflammatory effects and interferes with the growth of tumours. A recent University of California study also suggests that curcumin may also help the immune system clear the brain of amyloid beta, which forms the plaques found in Alzheimer's disease. Cayenne pepper contains capsaicin, which studies have linked to weight loss, arthritic pain relief and cardiovascular health. Ginger is known in Ayurvedic medicine as the "universal healer" and is believed to have anti-inflammatory properties that may make it effective in managing arthritis.

To watch a clip about inflammation support, scan the QR barcode above into your smart device or enter the following link into your browser: http://bit.ly/MAY1wl

Turmeric (*Curcuma longa*)				
			$	!
May help to prevent inflammation, cancer, elevated cholesterol and liver failure.	Modest scientific support.	Easy-to-swallow capsule or liquid. But even easier to eat more food using Indian spices!	Very affordable at less than $1/day.	"Likely Safe (NMCD).
16	14	18	18	16
Overall rating: 82%				

THE RETREAT OF FAT. THE ADVANCE OF MUSCLE.

In the previous chapter, we looked at the dire consequences of metabolic syndrome, an unhealthy ratio between body muscle and body fat. These consequences include type 2 diabetes, heart disease, various cancers and stroke—and clearly, a way to help prevent all of these from happening to you is to change that ratio in a positive way.

Weight Management

What the scale says is not a definitive assessment of your body's composition. Even after losing weight, you may still be significantly and dangerously overweight because the weight you lose may consist of too much muscle as well as fat. But by increasing lean muscle mass at the same time as losing fat tissue, you'll eventually achieve

To watch a clip about body composition, scan the QR barcode above into your smart device or enter the following link into your browser: http://bit.ly/QtHCwf

an optimal ratio. The ideal percent of muscle to fat should be about 75 to 80 percent muscle and between 20 and 25 percent fat for women, and 80 to 85 percent muscle or 10 to 15 percent fat in men. The higher your ratio of muscle to fat, the more calories your body will burn daily. In the sections following, I'll look at how we can achieve that by increasing our metabolic rate and, increasingly, our energy output through exercise and supplements.

IMPROVING OUR METABOLIC RATE

Knowing what we do about metabolic rate, it stands to reason that increasing that rate may be a more effective approach to weight loss (and thus health) than concentrating on controlling weight alone.

Here are a few key tips to optimize your metabolism. First, aim for total nutrition by using a multivitamin that is high in the B vitamins. Extra vitamins and minerals will help ensure your body gets the nutrition it needs, especially if you're avoiding certain foods, but more importantly because your body's metabolic processes won't work properly without micronutrients. Second, find a diet that fits you personally. There is now available SNP testing for variations in genes that are involved in inflammatory responses to food, and for response to exercise. Results of these tests can help guide weight management by predicting which combinations of diet and exercise will work best. In general, for long-term success, choose a healthy diet that you can stay with, but more importantly, increase foods that have been shown to boost metabolism. Interestingly, some of the spices we discussed as anti-inflammatory—curry, capsaicin and ginger, for example—can do just that. Try eating small meals five or six times per day to keep the metabolic fire stoked. Third, create a customized exercise plan. Aim to exercise in the morning and do the type of exercise you truly enjoy so that it is easier to stick to. Find activities that fit your personal style, fitness level and workout opportunities. It's common sense that exercise increases your metabolic rate. In Chapter Four we'll discuss staying well by staying fit.

When it comes to natural health products, many people are turning to pyruvate supplementation for a metabolic boost. Pyruvate is a substance naturally produced in the body during cellular metabolic processes. Combining exercise with 6 to 10 grams a day of this supplement may promote a beneficial speed-up of your metabolism. You may also want to try supplementing with 5-HTP (5-hydroxytryptophan), which we've encountered in earlier sections. Taking 200 to 400 mg of 5-HTP per day may help curb your appetite.

Not yet available in Canada (although coming soon to a health food store near you), the amino acid L-carnitine has been shown to be helpful for weight loss because of its role in fat metabolism. And green tea extracts, which we're hearing a lot about these days, have been shown to have positive effects on human metabolism.

To watch a clip about how to speed up your metabolism, scan the QR barcode above into your smart device or enter the following link into your browser: http://bit.ly/NQKApX

Gaining Muscle

It's now common knowledge that the numbers of Canadians who are at risk of metabolic syndrome has dramatically increased, mirroring a worldwide phenomenon. As a result of this growing awareness, many of us are making the effort to exercise regularly—walking, biking or joining a local gym or yoga class—while eating clean, sleeping well and keeping stress levels as low as possible. If you're among the converted, keep in mind that your routine should be one that doesn't injure you yet pushes your body to reap maximum results. A perfect choice might be a weight-bearing routine that achieves a full range of motion of muscles and includes stretching and effective warm-ups and cool-downs. The goal is to reach your personal potential and maybe lose that extra ten or twenty pounds.

So let's assume you're eating no refined, packaged, nutrient-devoid, processed garbage and you're exercising four times a week for a good, intense hour and you're sleeping well—a seven- or eight-hour minimum—and you've kept stressful factors relatively under control. You're doing all that but you're still working towards that optimal weight. Consider adding some natural health products to your routine. In the sections below, I recommend several that have the potential to support your workout regimen.

Workout Support

Your diet will be a key component in any exercise regimen. You can get off to a delightful start by spicing up whatever constitutes your daily diet with hot peppers. "What?" I hear you say. But researchers at Laval University in Quebec have found that eating hot peppers can speed up your metabolism and cool your cravings. Capsaicin (a chemical found in jalapeño and cayenne peppers) temporarily stimulates your body to release more hormones that speed up your metabolism and cause you to burn more calories. These studies found that people who ate spicy food tended to eat 30 percent less calories during the day. Most spices inhibit adipogenesis, that is, new fat cell formation, but also seem to decrease cravings and a preoccupation with the thought of food, at least when used by those who infrequently use spice.

Beyond the numerous benefits of a good diet, there are now natural health supplements on the market that can help you increase muscle mass.

The amino acid glutamine is the most abundant amino acid in the body and your muscles rely heavily on it to maintain size. Glutamine may also benefit the immune system. Double-blind trials have found that 81 percent of athletes given glutamine reported having no subsequent infection compared with 49 percent in the placebo group. And combining the amino acid arginine with glutamine and HMB (beta hydroxy-beta-methylbutyrate) may preserve lean body mass when dieting. You might also try 5 mg/1tsp of the amino acid L-glutamine in some freshly squeezed orange juice just prior to your workout.

L-carnitine is normally manufactured by the human body and has the ability to increase work capacity. The body needs the amino acids lysine and methionine, with vitamin C, iron, niacin and vitamin B6, to produce carnitine. Studies have found that L-carnitine improves certain measures of muscle physiology, in particular muscle's ability to convert stored fat to energy. Although not yet available in Canada, many athletes believe that L-carnitine improves their performance and appears to be a good supplement to take if you participate in endurance activities such as running. By transporting fatty acids into the mitochondria, L-carnitine can make exercise more productive, particularly for obese people.

To watch a clip that considers the power of tea for weight loss, scan the QR barcode above into your smart device or enter the following link into your browser: http://bit.ly/NsuWVZ

You might also look at conjugated linoleic acid (CLA) at 100 mg per ten pounds of body weight. Studies have shown that this safe, anti-carcinogenic fatty acid can play an effective

To watch a clip about how to speed up your metabolism, scan the QR barcode above into your smart device or enter the following link into your browser: http://bit.ly/NQKApX

role in reducing body fat and producing gains in muscle size and strength in weight-training men. These increases in muscle mass can in turn increase your metabolism.

Other studies have suggested that green tea extract boosts metabolism and may aid in weight loss. Its mood-enhancing ingredients have also been reported to contain anti-cancer properties and help prevent heart disease.

A note of caution, though: avoid supplements such as citrus aurantium and ephedrine that mess with your heart by increasing your heart rate.

Electrolytes as Supplements

Electrolyte-enriched products—including bottled waters, teas, juices, gels, tablets and bars—are often recommended for people who are doing exercise programs. But who needs them? Why? And when?

Electrolytes are molecules in the body—sodium, potassium, magnesium, chloride, calcium—and compounds that bind to them to create salts such as bicarbonates, phosphates and sulphates. Electrolyte molecules are positively or negatively charged, which allows them to carry electrical impulses that transmit nerve signals and contract muscles. They also maintain fluid levels and acid-base balance, making them indispensable for good health.

A normal diet usually provides more than enough electrolytes to meet the body's needs. But there are times when electrolytes from food alone may not be enough. For light exercise in moderate climates, replenishing water without electrolytes is sufficient for most people. But when temperatures rise or workouts are prolonged, more electrolytes may be lost through sweat than can be replenished with food alone. Sweating is the body's way of ridding itself of heat, but unfortunately this rids us of electrolytes too. Athletes training in hot climates are most likely to need electrolyte replacement. Muscle cramps are one hint that electrolytes may be running low when you're sweating a lot.

To watch a clip about electrolyte and pre-workout support, scan the QR barcode above into your smart device or enter the following link into your browser: http://bit.ly/MXzUnl

There are many natural health electrolyte replacement products, most providing sodium and potassium since these are lost in the largest quantities. (We only lose small amounts of magnesium.)

For healthy adults, sports drinks are most popular for electrolyte replacement, but if you're working out with weight loss in mind, watch the sugar content. You may not need the extra calories or the artificial colours and flavours.

Post-Workout Support

What is the best fat-burning workout? Simple. It's the one that exacts the highest metabolic cost, that is, burns the most calories.

Most folks think that simply exercising burns a lot of calories, but the truth is that we rarely burn that many calories *during* an exercise session. It's what happens *after* your workout that matters most.

EPOC stands for "excess post-exercise oxygen consumption" and refers to the fact that after cardiovascular training, the body continues its need for oxygen at a higher rate than normal. As a result, we burn calories at a higher rate during the twenty-three hours *following* a workout. Clearly, the higher the EPOC the greater the fat loss and, contrary to what you might think, the highest EPOC effect is associated with resistance training. Not the treadmill or the Stairmaster but *weight training*!

When you train with weights or push your body against gravity, you increase fat burning for the entire day. Try this workout if you want to give your metabolism a shot in the arm:

- Push-up x 10
- Lunge with shoulder press x 10
- Dumbbell row x 10
- Squats x 10

Use a controlled tempo: three seconds to lower the weight, no pause at the bottom and a quick-burst return to the starting position. Perform this sequence three times and use a weight that is challenging enough that the tenth repetition is quite difficult. This is also excellent cardiovascular training.

To watch a clip about post-workout support, scan the QR barcode above into your smart device or enter the following link into your browser: http://bit.ly/ME8CF3

We've already looked at the amino acid L-glutamine as an aid to increasing muscle mass. It also seems L-glutamine in some orange juice followed by a protein powder shake twenty minutes later can accelerate your post-workout recovery. Glutamine is the most abundant amino acid in the body and your muscles rely heavily on it to maintain size. And as a bonus, L-glutamine benefits your immune system.

Losing the Fat

As more and more people struggle to shed extra fat, many have contemplated weight-loss dietary supplements. The global weight-loss market reached an incredible $26 billion in 2009. To help you make wise choices and avoid falling prey to dietary supplement fraud, the United States Food and Drug Administration (FDA) recently released a "Consumer Update" to address the topic, and the Canadian Natural Health Product Directorate (NHPD) is regulating all products and their label claims.

When desperate to lose weight, many people will try almost anything—including a sketchy online supplement order. Not long ago, many supplements sold online and even many sold by reputable retailers were found to contain toxins and powerful drugs. Some "natural" diet products have been found to contain sibutramine (Meridia), a weight-loss medication removed from the market in 2010 because it increases risk of heart problems and stroke. Other FDA research has uncovered weight-loss supplements contaminated with seizure and blood pressure medications and even prescription drugs that were never approved at all.

Just remember that "caveat emptor" still applies in the supplement industry. When claims seem too good to be true, then trust your instinct. Products that promise quick action ("Lose 40 pounds in one month!") are marketed as having actions that are more powerful than recognized and approved weight-loss drugs or tout a revolutionary new scientific—yet proprietary—breakthrough should raise a red flag. These products may contain unapproved or potentially harmful ingredients, including prescription medications.

Here are a few tips that will help you make the most of any dietary supplement you decide to try.

- Talk to a well-qualified natural health practitioner or a doctor or dietitian who knows supplements.

- If you take prescription medications; if you have a heart condition, heart disease, diabetes, kidney disease or high blood pressure; or if you suffer from anxiety, depression or other mental health issues, do not use weight-loss supplements without your doctor's guidance. Some products can significantly worsen these conditions. You can reference my supplement–drug interactions guide here: http://www.wyldeabouthealth.com/healthnotes/us/assets/a-z-index/a-to-z-index-of-medicines/~default
- Always read labels. Be especially cautious with products manufactured in a foreign country, as many of these do not meet North American guidelines.
- Watch out for outrageous testimonials or claims.
- If you think you've had a bad reaction to a dietary supplement, notify the NHPD or FDA through their website or by phone. This is the only way to make sure harmful products are taken off the market. And make sure you also do this for prescription medication!

To watch a clip about weight management, scan the QR barcode above into your smart device or enter the following link into your browser: http://bit.ly/M6q48Y

Having raised the alarm, I'd like to mention some products that are worth investigating to see if they are right for you. One of my favourite combination supplements for effective weight loss—a product that has science to back up the label claim that it "aids in weight loss"—is conjugated linoleic acid (CLA) and epigallocatechin gallate (EGCG).

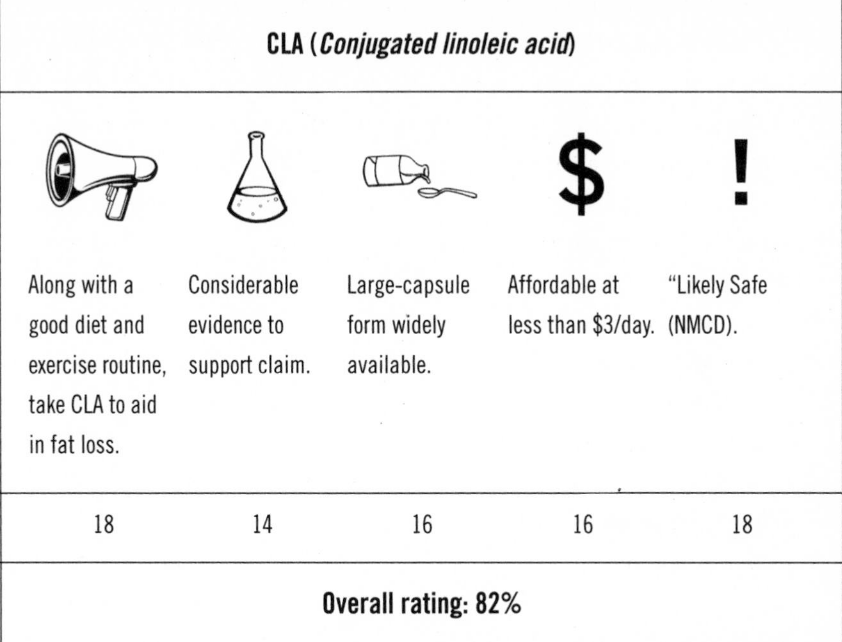

CLA (*Conjugated linoleic acid*)				
			$	!
Along with a good diet and exercise routine, take CLA to aid in fat loss.	Considerable evidence to support claim.	Large-capsule form widely available.	Affordable at less than $3/day.	"Likely Safe (NMCD).
18	14	16	16	18
Overall rating: 82%				

AMINO ACID THERAPY

Amino acid therapy is based on the theory that many symptoms and illnesses occur because the body is unable to manufacture the proper amino acid. This is in some respects similar to vitamin deficiency. By supplementing the body's normal supply of amino acids, symptoms and illnesses may be resolved.

Amino acids have been used in clinical tests to treat a variety of serious illnesses and conditions including: phenylketonuria (or PKU), epilepsy, hepatitis complications, lateral sclerosis, chronic pain, liver cancer, muscular dystrophy and hypertrophy of the prostate. There is also good evidence supporting the use of amino acid therapy to treat serious psychological disorders such as drug dependency, depression and anxiety.

Some health-care professionals may recommend taking only the eight essential amino acids, the ones your body obtains through diet. Some foods such as soy, garlic and some teas also contain amino acids. You may wish to incorporate more amino-rich foods into your diet, but you will achieve a much greater therapeutic result by taking a natural health product that offers truly supplemental levels of amino acids.

There is good scientific evidence that dietary supplementation with L-arginine, for example, may help people with coronary artery disease, angina or atherosclerosis, due to its effects on increasing or widening the blood vessels.

According to the A.P. John Institute for Cancer Research, controlled amino acid therapy combined with chemotherapy or used alone has reduced the burden of tumours in certain types of cancers and has improved patients' quality of life. Needless to say, effective treatment must be customized to each individual for optimal benefit.

THE ACID-BASE BALANCING ACT

In Chapter Two, we touched briefly on the importance of maintaining our bodies' correct acid-base balance. From improving physical and mental energy and increasing vitality, to turning on the cells that form strong bone, the health benefits of a proper acid-base balance are many.

How do we reach this most important benchmark? First, we need to cut down on our overly acidic diet. In general, however, I believe that an optimal diet of the sort discussed throughout this book, perhaps supplemented by one of the commercial "greens" concentrates, is likely to be an effective way to *buffer* the typical North American acidic diet. Scientists at leading universities throughout North America are continuing to understand that fruits and vegetables in high amounts—along with those "greens" formulas—exert such wide-ranging health benefits partly through their buffering of acid diets. Since pH is measured using a logarithmic scale whereby every point of pH represents a tenfold difference in acid load, any change at all in the direction of alkalinity, even a small one, is health promoting.

Finally, I wouldn't be doing my job if I didn't name some names. It's true that the "green" diet is a potent buffer against those foods that create an acidic bodily environment. But clearly it would also be beneficial to get to know specifically not only what foods are best in this respect, but what foods are *not* in our best interests in a fast-food culture that eats way too much of the wrong stuff. Scientifically, this comparison of foods is expressed as a number, the potential renal acid load of foods (PRAL), that is, how a food in question influences the pH of urine, which in turn is related to the pH environment of the body. We've encountered this measure already but it's not necessarily easy to determine intuitively. Lemons, for instant—obviously acidic—have an alkalizing effect in the body. The actual calculation is expressed as: PRAL = 0.49 Protein + 0.037 Phosphorus - 0.021 Potassium - 0.026 Magnesium - 0.013 Calcium.

We don't need to get into long and confusingly precise lists of foods and their PRAL values, though I encourage you to explore the fascinating subject of our body's pH. For us the key point is that adequate nutrition requires a balance of foods that have acidic and alkaline effects and *our diets consist of too many foods that acidify our body.* Let's close with some simple examples.

Foods Producing a Strong Alkaline Effect

Spinach
Celery
Dandelion
Endive, fresh
Green beans
Garlic
Leeks
Peas
Cayenne pepper
Cucumber
Sprouted chia seed
Watercress
Chives
Beet root

Carrots
Avocado
Lemon
Lima beans
Soybeans
Navy beans

Foods Producing a Strong Acidic Effect

White bread
Beef
Chicken
Eggs
Ocean fish
Pork
Veal
Hard cheese
Peanuts
Pistachios
Artificial sweeteners
Chocolate
Fructose
Ketchup
Mayonnaise
Soy sauce
Vinegar
Beer
Coffee
Liquor

To watch a clip about pH support, scan the QR barcode above into your smart device or enter the following link into your browser: http://bit.ly/MjFvWQ

I think the overall impression is obvious. Many popular foods are acidifying. We *need* those greens.

CHAPTER 4

STAYING HEALTHY: YOU DON'T HAVE TO FEEL BAD TO FEEL BETTER

We've looked so far at the contributions that integrative medicine can make to discovering how healthy we really are. And where we have reason to suspect a problem, we've looked at what we can do to put it right using the many products we generally identify as "natural." Now I want to close the circle by talking about how we can preserve that health as long as possible. We don't hope for physical immortality, but we do hope to remain sound and vigorous for as much of our life as possible. This means exploring the best ways to avoid the common problems we've discussed so far and the best plans for prevention. I want to talk about diet—there's always something new to say on that subject—and the supplements and lifestyle routines that are considered the best. I'm going to use the same seven categories I've used in the other chapters and for the same reason: these are the issues that come up again and again on my television shows and in meetings with my patients.

To use the metaphor of flight, you might say we've attained a comfortable altitude of well-being and now we want to level off and maintain our cruising speed. Come follow me!

1. THE IMMUNE SYSTEM IN BALANCE

FROM MUSHROOMS TO SEAWEED: THE ASIAN DIET SECRET

Our immune system's first line of defence is an evolutionarily older strategy. This is the so-called innate immune system—cells and mechanisms on guard against infection by other organisms but in a non-specific manner. Our innate immune system does not confer long-lasting or protective immunity.

"Adaptive immunity" is a newer and more "intelligent" system that is activated by the non-specific innate immune system. Adaptive immunity can recognize and remember specific pathogens and thereby mount stronger attacks each time the pathogen is encountered. It's also more intelligent in the sense that it prepares itself for future challenges. A truly healthy immune system is one that can fight off an infection quickly and effectively with a minimum of complications.

You'll remember cytokines, our messengers on the battlefield of the cellular war. It's really helpful to understand a

To watch a clip about immune support, scan the QR barcode above into your smart device or enter the following link into your browser: http://bit.ly/PBBKj3

bit about how these guys work because, if we do, we can adopt targeted nutrition regimens that reduce inflammation and create strength and balance in the immune system. And, as many modern studies show, one of the best ways of accomplishing this is eating more of what people in Asian cultures have traditionally eaten.

Allergies

As we've seen, allergic reactions are the result of a confused immune system. But we've come to recognize that algae and the related single-celled chlorella, which have been long used in traditional Chinese medicine, can quell an over-reactive immune system. We know that interleukin 5 (IL-5), a cytokine, stimulates white blood cells called B-lymphocytes that in turn stimulate the production of a protein immunoglobulin E (IgE), which is involved in allergy symptoms. It appears that algae and chlorella may inhibit antigen-induced production and so inhibit interleukin 5.

Cancer

Cancerous cells can eventually flourish when a key part of our immune army—the natural killer cells—aren't doing their job. Maitake mushrooms can increase natural killer activity since they and the maitake D-fraction prepared from them contains a type of polysaccharide (a large molecule formed by multiple sugar molecules linked together) called beta glucan. Beta glucan is believed to stimulate the immune system and activate certain cells and proteins that attack cancer, including macrophages, T-cells, natural killer cells and the cytokines IL-1 and IL-2 (interleukin-1 and -2).

Both algae and hijiki, a brown sea vegetable growing wild on rocky coastlines around Japan, Korea and China, may possess natural anti-cancer properties. Hijiki and algae may facilitate the release of the TNF-α from macrophages, the killer white blood cells. TNF stimulates the proliferation of B-lymphocytes and diminishes the supply of blood and oxygen to tumours.

Endogenous TNF possesses anti-angiogenesis properties that disrupt the tumour's ability to grow a blood supply.

Autoimmunity

Autoimmune diseases typically present an excess of symptoms related to inflammation.

Coconut oil, fish oils, flax seed oil and most nuts and seeds—all prominent in Asian diets—inhibit the production and release of inflammation. The mechanism may hinge on the way these oils inhibit the production of the protein interleukin-6; excessive IL-6 can lead to pro-inflammatory and autoimmune conditions.

Bacterial Infection

Bacteria and other microbes can multiply when our immune system is weakened. Barley grass, garlic and various mushrooms including enoki, reishi and maitake, all common in Asian diets, stimulate the immune system by enhancing the production of interleukin-2, which in turn stimulates the conversion of T-lymphocyte cells to natural killer lymphocytes that protect against microbial infection.

To watch a clip about infection and antiseptic support, scan the QR barcode above into your smart device or enter the following link into your browser: http://bit.ly/MAW1V8

Viral Infection

We're more vulnerable to viral infections when our immune defences are low. Spirulina (the microalgae usually available as green tablets), propolis (the resinous mixture that honeybees collect from tree buds and sap flows) and yogurt all have properties that increase the body's natural anti-viral defences by facilitating the release of interferon gamma (IFN-γ) from macrophage white blood cells. Interferon gamma stimulates the activity of macrophages, increases TNF activity and is crucial in inhibiting viral replication.

The epitome of health is not whether you get sick, but how *quickly* and *efficiently* your body is able to fight the infection and recover from it.

If you are getting sick no more than three or four times a year and the illness never complicates or lasts more than two or three days, then you are *staying healthy!*

SUPPLEMENTATION: MODULATING OUR IMMUNE SYSTEM

Immune *stimulation* is far different than immune *modulation*. Don't wait to get sick before you supplement your immune system, especially if you tend to get rundown and contract the common cold, flu or bacterial infections, perhaps because you travel frequently or are a parent of children in daycare. Of course, you'll want to fortify and balance your immune system. That's called *immunomodulation*.

A number of supplements are famous for their immunomodulation potency. Here are three I rate as the best:

AHCC

Active hexose correlated compound (AHCC) is an alpha-glucan-rich extract from the vegetative part of certain mushrooms like the Basidiomycota mushrooms, the family of the shiitake. It is in fact one of the world's most-researched immune supplements, with nearly a hundred supporting research studies. AHCC is considered the daily immune supplement of choice for those seeking to help their bodies fight the formation of abnormal cells and infections. It is a leading alternative cancer therapy used in hundreds of cancer clinics throughout Asia where it is also popular as a standard preventative regimen for all incoming patients to reduce the risk of hospital infections.

Plant Sterols and Sterolins

In Chapter Three, we saw how sterols are excellent for lowering cholesterol. But sterols, like most natural remedies, have multiple benefits and are also excellent at balancing immune activity. Sterol and sterolin nutrients occur in all plant life, and have been the subject of studies conducted in people with rheumatoid arthritis, HIV, general immune function, tuberculosis and stress-induced immune suppression. The results of these studies have been promising.

Vitamin D_3

Vitamin D_3, known as the "sunshine vitamin," is essential to life. Too many studies to mention in recent years have indicated that vitamin D_3 is a powerful immune modulator, and deficiency in D_3 has been linked to autoimmune disorders. Multiple sclerosis, for an example, is clearly an epidemiological issue—virtually non-existent at the equator but common in more northerly and southerly latitudes. The best source of D_3 is sunshine, but when sunshine is not an option, supplemental D_3 can help. Your doctor has likely already told you how important it is that you supplement with it and I'm telling you too. Regardless of where you live, it is important to get optimal doses of vitamin D if you want to avoid getting sick. Remember, optimal doses are not the same as minimum requirements. For many, optimal means 2,000 to 3,000 IU/day. Since pigmentation reduces vitamin D production in the skin, vitamin D insufficiency is more prevalent among African Americans and other dark-skinned individuals than among light-skinned people. Of course, getting tested to determine your body's current demand for D_3 is always important.

And finally, there is a fine balance to be struck between the use of direct sunlight to produce vitamin D and staying out of direct sunlight to avoid skin damage and the increased risk of skin cancers, especially the deadly melanoma. The stark truth is that there is no good argument for excessive sun exposure for most people with fairer skin. Dark-skinned people living in tropical climes are probably getting enough vitamin D without excessive risk from sun damage. Light-skinned people living at the same latitudes are at increased risk of sun damage. Conversely, dark-skinned people living far from the equator, where winters are longer and the sun's rays more inclined, are in greater danger of vitamin D insufficiency. Ironically, the same applies to their light-skinned neighbours who are trying to protect their skin with effective sunscreens. The common-sense conclusion: many people require vitamin D supplementation.

TOXIN-FREE LIVING

It's not possible to avoid environmental toxins. We all know that. *But* overexposure to toxins can do major damage to our immune system. The term "immunotoxicity" refers to an immune system overwhelmed by so many toxins that it can't function to protect you from invaders. In my clinical experience, immunotoxicity is usually the first problem that shows up in a patient's history, typically manifesting itself as allergies or asthma. Adults who for all their lives are "okay" and then suddenly experience allergy problems are especially suspect for immunotoxicity. They often have unusual reactions—they might suddenly feel they can't breathe—to something as innocuous as walking down the soap aisle in the grocery store. Chemical sensitivities are a common finding in people with immunotoxicity. Unrecognized damage to the immune system can even be responsible for chronic infections a person can't shake.

As we discussed in Chapter Two, toxins can be poisons produced even by our body's own processes. Toxins can occur in nature though manufactured sources—pesticides in our food, gas given off by a new carpet, chemicals in the water, that "new car" smell, toxic minerals used by industry and numerous other sources including prescription drugs—are generally the worst. Many toxins produced by petrochemicals (and those found in plastics) are xenoestrogens, meaning that they mimic estrogen in the body and contribute to hormone imbalance with subsequent immune suppression. Thousands of new chemicals are added each week to this chemical pile-up and our immunological intolerance to the modern environment is a serious worry.

The body is designed to detoxify itself, but when external sources of toxicity are added to the mix, those normal detoxification processes become overwhelmed. Our job has to be to significantly limit our exposure to toxins. Here are a few excellent places on the Internet that constitute tremendous databases that will help you do just that:

- To know your cosmetics and use only those that are safe: **http://www.ewg.org/skindeep**
- To learn to use alternatives to harmful chemicals in your home: **http://environmentaldefence.ca/campaigns/toxic-nation/alternatives-in-your-home**
- To familiarize yourself with what's beyond your home: the heavy metals in drinking water and contaminants in the air: **http://www.ewg.org/environment**

To watch a clip about the toxins in the home, scan the QR barcode above into your smart device or enter the following link into your browser: http://bit.ly/SR9ZmO

2. YOUR GUTS, YOUR GLORY

DIET: INCREASING YOUR FIBRE

We get fibre from fruits, vegetables, beans, legumes, whole grains, nuts and seeds. An intake of about 25 to 40 grams of fibre a day is linked to a reduced risk of developing heart disease, diabetes, high blood pressure, colon cancer and other intestinal disorders. A recent study in the *Archives of Internal Medicine* reports that eating an abundance of dietary fibre may lower the risk of an early death by as much as 22 percent. Our modern diet averages about ten grams a day. What can I say?

There are two types of fibre: soluble and insoluble. The soluble fibre passes into our bloodstream and works to balance blood sugar and reduce cholesterol and visceral fat. Insoluble fibre—what we often refer to as roughage—helps to maintain stool bulk, decreases our chances of falling victim to certain forms of cancer and helps keep intestinal bacterial colonies strong.

To maintain digestive and overall health, most of us need to significantly increase our intake of fibre. Rather than try to tell you exactly how many servings per day *you* need, let me instead define the ideal stool—the perfect poo. Once you achieve this, er, benchmark, you're getting enough fibre. How will you know? Simple. Once daily your bowel movement is a brief act and not a dreaded chore, you hear a swish like a good dive versus a belly flop and turn to a see a dark brown, S-shaped form in the toilet bowl. You finish off with only a small amount of toilet paper and a single wipe. Am I being clear?

Let me explain. An ideal bowel movement can be assessed by considering two main factors: frequency and consistency. To determine frequency, we'll use what I call the 3:3 rule of stool. It is unhealthy if you go more than three times a day but it is also unhealthy if you're not going at least once every three days. The actual transit time of your bowels—based on what you eat and when it comes out—should be approximately twenty-four hours. You'd like to time it, right? So much of this book is devoted to self-testing. Try eating a corn on the cob and taking note of the time elapsed between your swallowing the kernels and their reappearance in your stool. Take an average of three different times on three different days (leave a few days in between). That is your transit time. This test works as well as it does because we're not able to digest the skin on the kernels. If you're allergic to corn, try beets. A red stool in sight after a day is just right.

And, in case you were wondering why your stool is almost consistently brown, brown is the colour of bile, produced by the liver and administered through the gallbladder. Should the gallstones that we spoke about earlier block your bile duct, your stool lightens up drastically (occasionally turning pale grey) and you need to present yourself to the ER if the pain didn't already get you there.

Once you're regular, you'll want to do an audit on the quality and consistency of your stool. Ideally you want a fully formed, whole stool, a stool like a sausage with cracks. It should be slightly S-shaped, which represents the shape of your lower colon. Stool that is in separate hard lumps and is difficult to pass typically represents constipation and is of course not what you want. Shy stool is also a problem. The bowel movement is signalled by an ineffective urge to go and the stool is produced by pushing and straining for some time, though it may exhibit a decent form when it finally does come out. This may be a sign of inflammation in the colon. On the other extreme, a loose and sloppy stool is evidence of

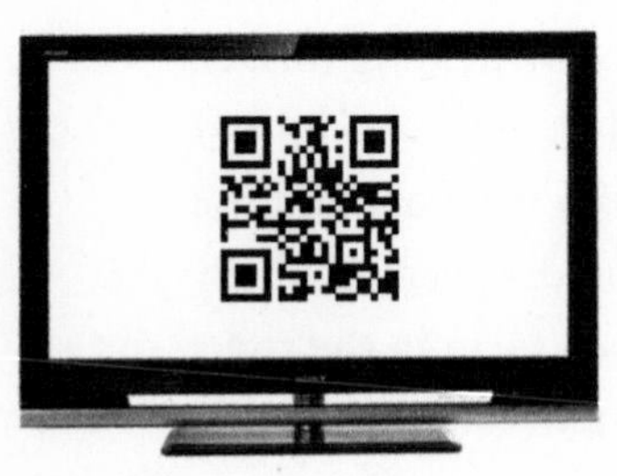

To watch a clip about the optimal bowel movement, scan the QR barcode above into your smart device or enter the following link into your browser: http://bit.ly/QgrPIF

the body rejecting something it is not happy with. It could also represent a bacterial overload or response to a virus. Frequent loose stools could be a sign of food intolerances. Diarrhea, an acute state, is watery, has no form, and is the body's "emergency evacuation" process.

Let's take a look, now, at the seven types of stool:

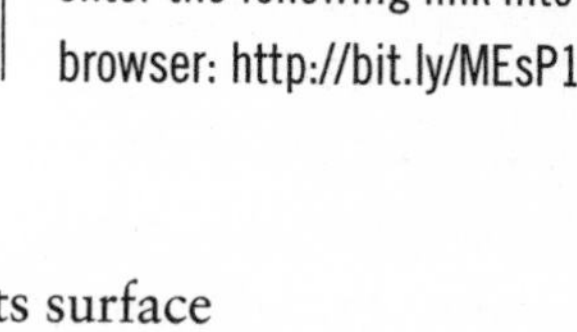

To watch a clip about intestinal support, scan the QR barcode above into your smart device or enter the following link into your browser: http://bit.ly/MEsP1f

Type 1: Hard dry lumps like walnuts that are difficult to pass
Type 2: Sausage-shaped and smooth
Type 3: A sausage but with cracks on its surface
Type 4: Like a sausage or snake, smooth and soft
Type 5: Soft blobs with clearcut edges (passed easily)
Type 6: Fluffy pieces with ragged edges, a mushy stool
Type 7: Water, no solid pieces. Entirely liquid

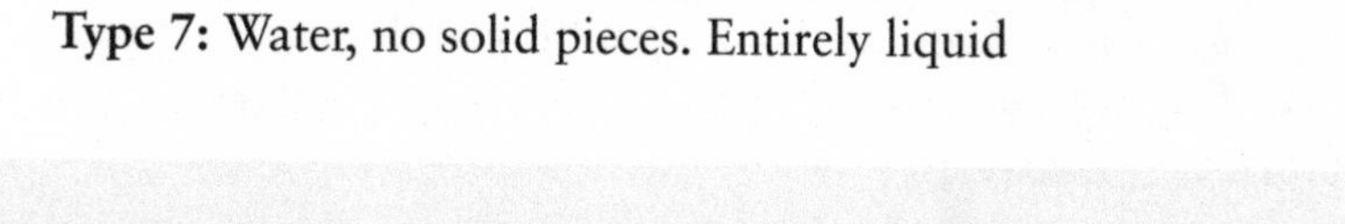

If you are having a bowel movement once daily and experience types 2 and 3 most often, you are *staying healthy!*

SUPPLEMENTATION: LIVER ENHANCEMENT AND INTESTINAL MAINTENANCE

The Quarterly Liver Enhancer

Glutathione is one of the most powerful antioxidants and natural detoxifiers in the human body. It is a very small protein composed of three amino acids: cysteine, glutamic acid and glycine. As it relates to our gut, there is some evidence that one of

To watch a clip about cleansing and natural detoxification support, scan the QR barcode above into your smart device or enter the following link into your browser: http://bit.ly/PBqeEj

its many roles is to prevent colon cancer, and the liver relies heavily on glutathione to remove impurities from your body. Glutathione slows down the aging process, detoxifies and improves liver function, strengthens the immune system, improves mental function and concentration, increases energy and improves heart and lung function. Sadly, since we constantly deal with more oxidative stress and toxins, our natural glutathione production drops about 1 percent every year.

There is little evidence that taking supplemental glutathione provides any benefit, so I'll share a recipe with you that can help your body make more of this powerful protein. As long as you get a go-ahead from your health-care provider, try supplementing with the following combination twice daily for two weeks every three months. The goal is to optimize your glutathione levels. I call it the "quarterly liver enhancement."

Supplement	Dose per 10 lbs body weight
L-glutamine	250 mg
N-acetyl cysteine (NAC)	50 mg
S-adenosyl methionine (SAM-e)	20 mg
alpha lipoic acid	15 mg
selenium	2.5 mcg
B complex	10 mg

The Monthly Pipe Cleaner

No matter how healthy we are, our intestines are a place where a lot of stuff can, um, go down. Polyps can harbour rogue cells that may one day turn cancerous and get the best of any of us, no matter how well we watch our diet. So once a month, I suggest you try this regular bowel cleanse:

In a ten-ounce glass of water, mix the following; consume at bedtime for three days.

- 1 tablespoon Bentonite Clay
- 1 tsp capryllic acid
- Open and mix in 1 capsule activated charcoal (between 300 and 600 mg)

For the next three days, consume broad-spectrum probiotics equivalent to 400 to 500 billion cells/dose.

LIFESTYLE: CHEWING, MIXING AND MOVING

You've probably heard that we all need to breathe more slowly and deeply. You may have also heard we need to slow down on our eating. I would tend to agree with both, but when it comes to eating, how slow is slow? How many times are we really supposed to chew?

Digestion begins in the mouth. The act of mastication tells the rest of your gastrointestinal system to begin the digestive process. There is no exact measure of how many clenches of your jaw you need to perform before you can swallow without worrying about your health. I advise all my patients with chronic indigestion to—among other things—chew until whatever is in your mouth turns to soup—then swallow. Your objective is to blend your saliva with your food because it's saliva that contains the enzyme amylase, whose function it is to begin the breakdown of carbohydrates. Interestingly, the carbohydrates in your food also give your immune system—and more specifically the mucous associated lymphoid tissue (MALT)—a heads-up as to what's in your mouth. For that reason alone, we should try to honour the eating process rather than mindlessly wolfing down our food. Mindful eating is half as much, twice as long! We need to take fifteen seconds or so to be appreciative of the food we have, perhaps take a few deep breaths to relax and allow our digestive system to work better. Otherwise it tends to shut down when we're stressed and on the go.

When you chew your food to liquid you can look forward to experiencing better digestion. Chewing breaks food into smaller particles and increases the surface area. You risk incomplete digestion by swallowing pieces—with bloating, gas and possible bacterial overgrowth in the gut. And of course the longer it takes to eat, the more efficient the message to the brain that you're full. Your blood sugar will be better balanced and, quite simply, you'll eat less because it takes more time. Finally, if nothing else persuades you, chewing better means we enjoy our food more. The flavours wash over our palate, satisfying our hunger more quickly and helping us maintain a healthy weight.

If you're chewing your food until you can no longer identify what you're eating by its texture, then you are *staying healthy!*

3. LIBIDO FOR LIFE

DIET: APHRODISIAC FOODS

Love in all its forms does receive a certain amount of scientific attention. Clinical sexologists are professionals who help clients gain or return to the sexual functioning they desire, and their research and clinical experience suggests that food—in particular the smell, taste and appearance of certain foods—can have potent aphrodisiac effects.

Food, it seems, can put you in the mood for love and even improve your pitch. In fact, specific foods appear to be appropriate at each stage of the courting process and applying this knowledge can enhance these effects. Enough to make your mouth water, right?

It's not difficult to believe that various nutrients and substances affect the body physiologically and that these effects differ according to the stage of the sexual or mating process. Certain foods lower inhibitions, some get the blood flowing directly to the genitalia, and others release happy hormones that can increase your self-confidence, lower your inhibitions and make you a more effective flirt.

Chili peppers. Somehow that makes sense, doesn't it? Chilis and other spicy foods get the heart pumping and induce sweating, releasing pheromones and increasing blood flow.

Bananas have long been known to contain neurochemicals that have a mood-lifting and confidence-lifting effect.

Fish. Foods rich in protein contain a large amino acid called tryptophan that helps us to produce serotonin, our brain's feel-good hormone. Omega-3 fats found in fish also help to increase blood flow, which all agree is important for a healthy sex life. Another salted herring, my dear?

Pumpkin seeds. Low levels of zinc could be to blame for a loss of sexual vitality—and pumpkin seeds are rich in zinc. Try adding pumpkin seeds to salads and even spread pumpkin seed butter on your morning toast to get your daily dose.

Ginger is known to increase blood flow to the genitals in both men and women.

Chocolate. Along with its jolt of caffeine, chocolate is rich in romantic associations.

Arugula is not just the lettuce alternative that separates you from the hoi polloi. Revered through history by Europeans as an aphrodisiac food and general clearer of the mind, its rich supply of vitamins A and C helps to put the body in its sexual prime.

When you're ready to seduce or be seduced, aphrodisiac foods can help trigger the release of sex hormones such as testosterone, provide a quick energy boost and increase blood flow to the relevant parts. But they can also create a visual stimulation. Experts say eating foods that look like the genitalia, such as oysters, fresh figs or carrots can help accomplish this.

The one thing *all* these foods have in common is that they also improve heart health, but then again, so does the act of sex itself. In a study published in the *Journal of Epidemiology and Community Health*, researchers found that having sex twice or more a week reduced the risk of fatal heart attack by half for men, compared with those who had sex less than once a month. But what about the sudden exertion of sex for older men? Other scientists followed 914 men for twenty years and found that greater frequency of sex was *not* associated with stroke.

More oysters, anyone?

To watch a clip about sexual support, scan the QR barcode above into your smart device or enter the following link into your browser: http://bit.ly/MEC4ic

SUPPLEMENTATION: THE OPTIMIZERS

A 2011 study suggests that fenugreek—an herb perhaps best known for its support in type 2 diabetes and for helping breast milk flow in women—may increase libido in men. Fenugreek is native to India and northern Africa. The study included sixty healthy men between the ages of twenty-five and fifty-two, none of whom had erectile dysfunction at the start of the trial.

They were randomly assigned to receive either 600 milligrams of fenugreek or a placebo daily for six weeks. The men answered questions about their sex drive and quality of life. Findings showed that fenugreek improved libido and quality of sexual performance compared to the placebo. Additionally, fenugreek was associated with improvements in overall quality of life and did not affect mood or sleep. Hormones such as prolactin and testosterone levels also remained within the normal range, suggesting a significant positive effect on the physiological aspects of libido in these men.

Still, my favourite sexual optimizer is maca root. Maca is a vegetable that has been cultivated as a root crop for at least two thousand years and is found wild in Peru and Argentina. It is sold in powdered supplement form and is also referred to as Peruvian ginseng, although it is not closely related to ginseng. Traditionally, it has also been used to relieve stress, as an aphrodisiac, and for fertility enhancement in both males and females. It is also purported to boost energy, balance hormones and enhance sexual performance. What's not to love about maca?

LIFESTYLE: MORE SEX

Having more sex sounds like it wouldn't be difficult, but in fact it can be, given the time constraints that contemporary lifestyles place on us. But in my view, sex is very much like exercise: you don't have the time *not* to engage! Regular sex is not only going to benefit your overall health and prevent disease, but twice or so per week helps to reduce stress. According to researchers from Scotland in a study published in *Biological Psychology,* a huge health benefit of sex is lower blood pressure and overall stress reduction. This group studied twenty-four women and twenty-two men who kept records of their sexual activity. Then the researchers subjected them to stressful situations such as speaking in public and doing verbal arithmetic and noted their blood pressure response to these stresses. Those who had had intercourse had better responses to stress than those who engaged in other sexual behaviours or abstained.

Regular sex also boosts your immune system. In other words, good sexual health may mean better physical health. Having sex once or twice a week has been linked with higher levels of an antibody called immunoglobulin A (IgA) which can protect you from getting colds and other infections. But, having sex too often may not be as effective. Like anything else, moderation is key. Scientists at Wilkes University in Wilkes in northeastern Pennsylvania studied 112 college students who reported the frequency of sex they had. Those who reported having sex once or twice a week had higher levels of IgA than those in the other three groups, who reported being abstinent, having sex less than once a week or having sex three or more times weekly. Of course, who knows if they were all telling the truth?

It may seem intuitive that sex is also a bit of a workout and who couldn't do with the additional caloric burn? But who knew that if you had sex in the above prescribed frequency you'd regularly burn approximately 4,000 to 5,000 calories or more monthly. That is more than enough to lose a pound or two depending on how vigorously you approach the project. Furthermore, as the hormone oxytocin surges during sex, endorphins increase and any minor pain you may be experiencing declines. So if your partner says, "I have a headache," you can provide assurances that you know exactly how to get rid of it. Oxytocin also improves sleep and of course getting enough sleep has been linked with preventing a host of other things such as obesity and elevated blood pressure.

Where it might be easy to believe that sex prevents heart disease, increases feel-good hormones, promotes a pain-free environment in the body and improves sleep, who would have imagined it could possibly reduce the risk of prostate cancer? It turns out that frequent ejaculations, especially in men in their twenties, may reduce the risk of prostate cancer later in life. A study by Australian researchers reported in the *British Journal of Urology International* found that men who had five or more ejaculations weekly while in their twenties later experienced a risk of getting prostate cancer that was reduced by a third. Another study reported in the *Journal of the American Medical Association* found that frequent ejaculations, twenty-one or more a month, were linked to lower prostate cancer risk in older men.

If you're getting lucky at least twice weekly, you're also *staying healthy!*

4. CHANGES OF HEART

DIET: GROW AND EAT AN ORGANIC RAINBOW

You already know what I'm going to say, right? Fruits and vegetables are high in antioxidants, folic acid, fibre and potassium—nutrients that help prevent heart disease. Most are also high in other vital nutrients and low in calories. They keep you feeling full and help you avoid eating those high-fat foods that aren't heart-healthy. For optimal heart health, choose fruits and vegetables that are fresh, organic and all the colours of the rainbow.

Many people ask me if organic is worth the extra expense. When I'm asked this question, I sometimes respond, "Is your health worth it?" But as a reader you'll want more than that. We first need to define what we mean by "organic." Organic farming relies on crop rotation, green manure, compost and biological pest control to maintain soil productivity and control pests on a farm. Organic farming excludes or strictly limits the use of manufactured fertilizers, pesticides (which include herbicides, insecticides and fungicides), plant-growth regulators such as hormones, livestock antibiotics, food additives and genetically modified organisms. Research has shown that *acute* pesticide exposure can cause heart disease but a study at Uppsala University in Sweden has recently found that chronic low-dose exposure to organochlorine pesticides may pose a risk for the development of atherosclerosis, which can lead to heart disease. My advice, given the current level of understanding? Spending a few extra bucks to buy organic is probably worth it.

According to Canadian organic standards, food products and agricultural products, including livestock and livestock feed, can only be referred to as organic if the farm they come from uses methods that aim to reduce harmful effects on the environment. This can be achieved using several methods for the nurturing of biodiversity, including planting a variety of crops to attract "good" insects and deal naturally with weeds, disease and pests. It may also entail rotating crops from season to season to avoid a buildup of certain kinds of pests or the depletion of certain nutrients in the soil.

Under the same standards, products that contain multiple ingredients (e.g., salsa) can only be labelled "organic" if at least 95 percent of the content is organic. Those that don't qualify but have more than 70 percent organic content can mention the percentage on their primary labelling. Products with less than 70 percent organic content can only refer to organic content in their ingredients list.

Organic farming does not allow for genetic engineering, certain kinds of fertilizers, certain forms of irradiation (like X-rays, typically used to reduce harmful bacteria and increase shelf life), synthetic pesticides and growth regulators, food additives like sulphates, nitrates and nitrites, the use of antibiotics or anti-parasite medication in animals (though there are some exceptions), or the cloning of animals and their offspring.

To ascertain whether a product is organic, look for an official certification on the label, usually in the form of a stamp of approval from the certifiers. For example, the United States Department of Agriculture (USDA) seal is acceptable, and the Canadian Food Inspection Agency (CFIA) stamp of approval is even better, because Canada has some of the highest standards in the world. Consumers can now rest assured that foods carrying this new CFIA logo meet organic requirements. If you want to make absolutely sure food labelled organic really is organic, check out the CFIA website at http://www.inspection.gc.ca/english/fssa/orgbio/orgbioe.shtml.

Must we *always* eat organic—100 percent of the time—to stay healthy? Not necessarily. If you haven't already met them, let me introduce you to the "Clean 15." Fifteen fruits and veggies have been found to have the lowest pesticide load and consequently are the safest conventionally grown crops to consume from the standpoint of pesticide contamination. They are: onions, avocados, sweet corn, pineapples, mangoes, sweet peas, asparagus, kiwi, cabbage, eggplant, domestic cantaloupe, watermelon, grapefruit, sweet potatoes and honeydew melon. Then there are the "Dirty Dozen" fruits and veggies, which have the highest pesticide load, making it most important to buy the organic versions or to grow them organically yourself. They include: celery, peaches, strawberries, apples, blueberries, nectarines, sweet bell peppers, spinach, collard greens/kale, cherries, potatoes and grapes, particularly imported grapes.

So, when and if you can afford it, my advice is to always buy organic if the produce in question isn't among the "Clean 15." But either way, trumping the importance of pesticide contamination and organic certification is the necessity of eating at least 7 to 10 half-cup servings of fruits and vegetables *every* day.

Which fruits and vegetables are most important and for what reason? This is where "eating a rainbow" comes in.

Red foods—cherries, red/pink grapefruit, cranberries, pomegranate, red grapes, strawberries, watermelon, beets, red onions, red pepper, red potatoes and tomatoes—contain lots of lycopene, which is excellent as protection against various cancers including prostate cancer.

Orange and yellow foods—squash, turmeric, cumin, apricots, grapefruit, mango, papaya, pineapple, carrot, yellow pepper, sweet potato/yam, lemons and mustard—contain many carotenoids, limonene and bioflavonoids that potently strengthen your immune system.

Green foods—avocado, green apples, kiwi, lime, green pears, artichokes, asparagus, broccoli, Brussels sprouts, green beans, green pepper and zucchini—contain lutein and indoles for vision and protect against various estrogen-related cancers.

To watch a clip about eating a rainbow of foods for optimal health, scan the QR barcode above into your smart device or enter the following link into your browser: http://bit.ly/OVrMED

Blue and purple foods—blueberry, eggplant, spanish onions, plums and acai berry—contain anthocyanins, incredible for cardiovascular health.

So if eating organic is necessary most of the time, eating a rainbow is absolutely crucial to your good health. And while we're at it, eating food grown locally tastes better and is better for you, is free of genetically modified organisms (GMOs) free, builds the local economy and supports a clean environment. So my challenge to you is this: eat, grow and enjoy a rainbow of fruits and vegetables every day. I challenge you to grow your very *own* rainbow, all organic, in your own backyard.

Your Garden

There is nothing more local than food from your own backyard. If you aren't doing it already and are unsure where to start, here's a short lesson on constructing a vegetable rainbow: red tomatoes, orange carrots, yellow peppers, green Swiss chard and purple beets.

Start with a plan and start early in the season. With organic vegetables, many varieties can only be grown from seed. For our rainbow selection, you'll want to start the tomatoes and peppers inside around the end of March. The beets, carrots and Swiss chard can be sown right into containers outside towards the end of May.

Starting inside from seed. Head to your local garden centre to pick up supplies. For novice gardeners, talk to them about your plans and have someone show you the equipment. First, choose your organic seeds according to your tastes and available growing conditions (light, space, etc.). Keep the seed packets or stick tags so you know when to harvest and what you planted. Then, pick up a seeding tray with a clear plastic dome. For the soil, you want a certified-organic seeding mix for edibles (as an example, manufacturers like Fafard and Premier Tech have third-party certified-organic mixes). Pick up a few small plastic pots for transplanting your seedlings later on. At home find a warm, sunny place for your seeding tray. For detailed instructions on planting your seeds I like to reference www.burpee.com/gygg. The seeds will germinate within a few weeks and you'll need to water regularly. Once the seedlings are 2 to 3 inches high, transplant them into larger individual growing pots. Fill the pots with soil and press down with your thumb to create a hole. Gently remove the seedlings from the cell packs, place them in the indentation and compress the soil around them. Continue to water the plants, keeping the soil moist but not wet.

Choosing your containers. Whenever it's planting season in your neck of the woods, you'll want to pick up outdoor containers. It's best to choose something rectangular to maximize the space for your veggies. It's also a good idea to plant your tomatoes in a separate round container due to their size. Make sure your containers have holes for drainage at the bottom. If they don't, drill three or four holes before filling them with soil.

Planting your seedlings and sowing seed. Once the risk of frost has passed in your area—check with your local garden centre for exact timing as this is very important—it's time to plant your tomato and pepper plants and sow the seeds for your carrots, beets and Swiss chard. Pick a location with as much afternoon sun as possible and fill your containers with the organic soil mix and compress gently. Plant your beets, carrots and Swiss chard in rows according to the package instructions. If you are planting more than one pepper plant, space them 2 feet apart. Plant 3 or 4 tomato plants on the perimeter of the circular pot, ideally about a foot apart. Tomatoes will need to be trained to grow up and there are many ways to do this so ask your local garden centre for options.

Summer maintenance. You'll need to water and fertilize your vegetables throughout the summer. Organic and natural fertilizers from manures and composts are of course preferred to chemicals. If you buy organic fertilizer preparations, not having a horse on hand, follow the package directions and water regularly; in the heat of the summer this may mean daily. You may need to prune the tomatoes, but the rest of the vegetables should be pretty maintenance free.

Harvest according to the package indications and enjoy the incomparable taste of your own organic fresh vegetables.

If you're eating 7 to 10 servings of rainbow-coloured organic fruits and vegetables every single day, you are *staying healthy!* Bonus if they're your own!

SUPPLEMENTATION: ANTIOXIDANT ARMOUR

In Chapters Two and Three, we met the destructive oxygen molecules known as free radicals. If you read my previous book, *The Antioxidant Prescription*, you got a sort of crash course in the science of oxidative stress. Here, I want to look briefly at the role of free radicals in heart disease.

When we think of heart disease, we're most likely to think of heart attacks, with the acute scenario of chest pain and often fatal consequences. But true heart disease starts well before the first symptoms are ever felt. Along with aging comes some degree of "hardening" of the arteries—as natural as wrinkles and sags—but *serious heart disease is not a natural consequence of aging.*

Let's look at this process by which the arteries age. At the beginning, free radicals attack the lining of the inside of an artery. If the interior lining of the artery is repeatedly injured, the body's natural response is to deposit cholesterol plaque at the site of the injury, much like putting little Band-Aids on superficial wounds. If there is too much low-density lipoprotein (LDL)—also known as "bad" cholesterol—in the system, the body may not know when to stop applying the Band-Aids. The plaque deposits grow and when they clog heart arteries, the result is the pain of restricted blood supply to the heart we know as angina. If plaque eventually breaks away to block a critical heart artery, or more commonly if the plaque develops a crack that initiates clot formation, crossing the artery completely, well, that's a heart attack.

So given that some of this artery damage is inevitable with age, why do I say that heart *disease* is not inevitable? First, because a preponderance of free radicals, with their ability to mediate artery damage, and LDL, which contributes to ongoing plaque formation, is to some degree in our control. And as I discussed in *The Antioxidant Prescription*, most of the damage to heart muscle inflicted by a heart attack is caused at a later stage, by a burst of free radicals *after* the blood flow is resumed, very similar to the way a stroke inflicts such dire effects on the brain. Those unfortunate enough to experience a stroke but fortunate enough to be taking antioxidants will always fare better in recovery. One free radical in particular, nitric oxide, may play a central role in this destruction (and one antioxidant, vitamin E, may play a key role in cleaning up the damage).

Yet nitric oxide—a free radical, remember—is essential for normal blood circulation. And the oft-misunderstood cholesterol is not all bad either: it's crucial to the functioning of our hormones, our immune system and the artery-repair system. Clearly, it's balance we require.

There are a number of supplements that can help us maintain the balance that our hearts and arteries depend on. The top three heart-healthy supplements are: CoQ10, pycnogenol and omega-3 essential fatty acids. Each of these can benefit anyone.

Coenzyme Q10 (CoQ10) is also called ubiquinone, a name that signifies its ubiquitousness—that is, widespread distribution—in the human body. CoQ10 is a powerful protective antioxidant used by the body to transform food into adenosine triphosphate (ATP), the energy on which the body runs. CoQ10 is particularly concentrated in the heart, where it contributes to that organ's energy-making mechanisms. CoQ10 can bring multiple benefits. Those with angina may experience greater ability to exercise without chest pain. CoQ10 may effect a significant lowering of blood pressure. Supplementation has been shown to benefit even trained athletes. Most people looking to thwart heart disease would do well to take 100 mg of the ubiquinol form daily with food.

To watch a clip about antioxidant support, scan the QR barcode above into your smart device or enter the following link into your browser: http://bit.ly/OXs15J

Pycnogenol is also an antioxidant. It comes from an extract of the bark of the French maritime pine, which grows along the Atlantic coast of southwestern France. It has been shown to reduce systolic blood pressure in people with mild hypertension, it may slow the progression of retinopathy and improve vision, and it can improve some measure of memory.

But the powerhouse panacea prevention pill (to the extent that there is one) is the omega-3. Omega-3 fats have gained a huge reputation over the last decade for contributing to the improvement of human health in many ways. Docosahexaenoic acid (DHA) and eicosapentaenoic acid (EPA) are the important omega-3s to know. This supplement is key for heart health as it is able to mitigate the all too often silent inflammation that can eventually cause damage to your arteries. A downside to this supernutrient, however, is that its primary source is fish, and global fisheries have largely been mismanaged over the past century. As a result, omega-3-rich fish such as cod, salmon, tuna and shark are threatened by overfishing. Our oceans have meanwhile become polluted, which makes heavy consumption of many fish a significant source of known carcinogens including mercury, PCBs and dioxins. Recent research shows that there is no safe level of mercury. To overcome the risk of these contaminants, several brands of fish oil supplements have had to purify the oil to create a safe and convenient source of omega-3s.

The most significant threat to global fisheries is the world's demand for meat. Farmed fish, cattle, poultry and pigs are fed a diet of fish meal and fish oil. Catching fish and rendering it to fish meal for the sole purpose of feeding other animals is known to be an ecologically unsound practice. For instance, it takes four pounds of fish meal to grow one pound of farmed salmon. Ludicrous.

The health hazards of a diet high in animal protein have been well documented. However, the most significant health hazard may be the effect it will have on future supplies of fish, including the fish oil supplements. To address this growing environmental concern some companies are starting to develop what may become the new "fish oil"—and it isn't even from fish. These plant equivalents to fish oil feature a combination of omega-3 sources that provide the body with the same benefits as do fish oils. Not that this is news. We've long known that common plants, grains, nuts and seeds, including those of flax, hemp, pumpkin, borage and canola are sources of omega-3. They differ from fish sources, however, in that they provide us with omega-3 fats in a form called ALA, whereas fish provide the bioactive forms EPA and DHA. The human body can convert ALA to EPA and DHA but the rate of this conversion is very low. Plant sources are also too heavily weighted to omega-6 and omega-9 oils and most of us already get excessive levels of these in our diets.

What can we do to end this frustrating cycle of nutritional shortage? Here is something you may not know: omega-3 constituents EPA and DHA are not exclusive to fish oils. The fish ultimately get the DHA from their consumption of algae, and DHA-rich algae can be grown in large tanks similar to the way beer is made. Whereas the yeast produce alcohol, the algae produce DHA.

Ah, but what about EPA, the other critical omega-3 oil from fish? Recently, developers of nutritional supplements have begun introducing a plant called "echium," native to many parts of the world and often thought of as a "weed." "Weeds," as everyone knows, grow extremely efficiently and do not generally require the use of pesticides, herbicides or fertilizers. Echium is a rare source of the omega-3 stearidonic acid (SDA). Whereas the omega-3 ALA (found, for example, in flax) converts poorly to EPA, the omega-3 SDA (found in echium) converts efficiently and rapidly to EPA. Combined with algae-produced DHA, we have an omega-3 supplement with the potency of fish oil.

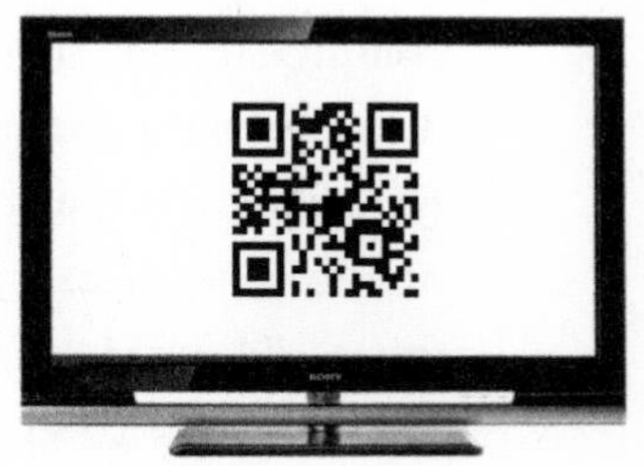

To watch a clip about omega-3 essential fatty acids, scan the QR barcode above into your smart device or enter the following link into your browser: http://bit.ly/MXakPG

So it looks as though our efforts to stay healthy may receive a further boost from the modern natural products industry, in this case a sustainable, low-energy replacement for fish oil—and one without any possibility of "BP seasoning" courtesy of the latest oil spill. How's that for a change of heart?

LIFESTYLE: TICKER TRAINING

There are libraries of books dedicated to improving heart health through exercise, so I won't try to discuss that type of training here. But there's another type of training for your heart and body—optimal heart-rate variability—that I do want to talk about.

Optimal heart-rate variability is about mindfulness and biofeedback. Simply put, the heart and brain maintain a continuous two-way dialogue, each influencing the other's functioning, and once you learn how to optimize your heartbeat you can in turn optimize your thoughts (and vice versa). The signals the heart sends to the brain can influence perception, emotional processing and higher cognitive functions. Neurocardiology researchers call this circuit the "heart brain."

The Institute of HeartMath (IHM) is an internationally recognized non-profit research and education organization dedicated to helping people of all ages reduce stress, self-regulate emotions and build energy and resilience for healthy, happy lives. IHM conducts ongoing research into heart-rate variability (HRV), a measure of the naturally occurring beat-to-beat changes in heart rate. HRV analysis is a powerful, non-invasive measure of autonomic nervous system function and an indicator of neurocardiac fitness. HeartMath has published research demonstrating how HRV varies with age and gender and on the use of HRV analyses to assess alterations in autonomic function in many conditions including panic disorder and chronic fatigue. Their studies using HeartMath techniques and technology have been published in many peer-reviewed journals including the *American Journal of Cardiology,* the *Harvard Business Review* and the *Journal of Alternative and Complementary Medicine.*

One of the technologies the IHM has employed with resounding success is biofeedback using a device called the "emWave." (Full disclosure: I use this myself, but I do not represent the company or receive any payments from them.) Biofeedback has been a prominent tool used for decades to track sensory data and provide a visual display of how stressors affect many bodily functions such as blood pressure, temperature and heart rate. Biofeedback measures your physiological response to stress. Using the emWave as a biofeedback device, you can learn how to prevent the negative effects stress may have on your body. The heart communicates via electromagnetic signals (EKG) that can be measured and interpreted by your doctor. But now similar technology is available to private individuals.

I've had the pleasure of speaking with Dr. Rollin McCraty who is a Ph.D. and the director of research at the Institute of HeartMath. He describes the emWave2 as an advanced heart rate monitor that displays your heart's rhythm, which in turn reflects your emotional state and helps you learn how to shift into an optimal state during stressful times.

The HeartMath system offers scientifically based and highly effective solutions for increasing overall performance by reducing stress, anxiety, depression and sleeplessness. The tools and techniques of this HeartMath system are based on over seventeen years of scientific research on the psychophysiology of stress, emotions and the interactions between the heart and brain. Most of us have been taught in school that the heart is constantly responding to "orders" sent by the brain in the form of neural signals. However, it is not commonly known that the heart actually sends more signals to the brain than the brain sends to the heart! Not only does the heart respond to the brain, but the brain continuously responds to the heart. Moreover, these heart signals have a significant effect on brain function influencing emotional processing as well as higher cognitive faculties such as attention, perception, memory and problem-solving.

To watch a clip about the Institute of HeartMath`s emWave, scan the QR barcode above into your smart device or enter the following link into your browser: http://bit.ly/Okg1cB

Research has demonstrated that different patterns of heart activity (which accompany different emotional states) have distinct effects on cognitive and emotional function. Through the use of biofeedback (and a device such as the emWave2), you can completely transform your response to stress and quickly rebalance your mind, body and emotions while increasing overall brain function. You will decrease stress and any environment-induced burnout that you may experience in your everyday life. Talk about a change of heart!

If you're eating an organic rainbow, taking your antioxidants and omega-3s and practising heart-healthy biofeedback, you are *staying healthy!*

5. MIND YOUR OWN BRAIN

THE BRAIN DIET

Nutritional neuroscience is one of the hottest topics in medicine today. There've been a lot of studies over the last few decades that demonstrate a strong correlation between nutrition and neurological function, cognition, and on brain-related conditions both psychiatric and psychological.

Food choices we made—or our parents made for us—throughout our lives and in particular during pregnancy, lactation and early childhood appear to have direct and long-term consequences on our mood, intelligence and behaviour. But it doesn't stop there. Our dietary choices throughout adulthood have a direct impact on our brainpower. Eating more herbs and spices, for example, can increase blood flow to the brain and with that comes oxygen. With oxygen comes brainpower and memory. Eating the *wrong* foods can gum up the arteries that supply the brain with blood, nutrients and oxygen and the result can be the exact opposite. Indeed, recent research suggests that our ever-expanding waistlines may be causing our brains to shrink—literally. Inflammation and free radicals that ramp up in the body as a consequence of eating the wrong foods appear to play a role as underlying nutritional causes for depression, anxiety, multiple sclerosis, Parkinson's, Alzheimer's, migraine headaches, ADHD and a whole lot more.

Carbohydrates, amino acids, fats, vitamins, antioxidants and essential fatty acids are all essential requirements for brain structure and function. Complex carbohydrates and vitamins fuel the brain, amino acids enable the brain's internal communications, fats make up the structure of the brain, and antioxidants protect the brain. What we now know about food and nutrition and how it can impact brain health was unimaginable only a few years ago.

Our brains are responsible for intelligence, memory, emotion, attention, consciousness—in fact, a whole lot of what we think of as ourselves. In the face of this new research, we have to consider that slight deficiencies in certain nutrients such as omega-3 fatty acids can influence all of these factors, while increasing our chances of depression and cognitive disorders such as Alzheimer's disease. Clinical studies in prisons in the United States and the United Kingdom have shown decreased acts of violence among subjects who received fish oil and multivitamins in their diet and this was accompanied by improved test scores in those with learning disorders, and improved mood scores in those with depression. Many other studies, including one done in 2005 reported in the *European Journal of Clinical Investigation*, have shown that taking fish oil supplements improved cognitive functioning and mood scores in otherwise healthy adults.

After our discussion in the previous section, you won't be surprised to discover that what is good for the heart is good for the brain. A heart-healthy diet and a brain-healthy diet both manage oxidative stress—that is, free radical generation—and inflammation. Dietary antioxidants from deeply coloured fruits and vegetables protect the blood vessel walls, and omega-3 essential fats dampen down the inflammation process that is

To watch a clip about nervous system support, scan the QR barcode above into your smart device or enter the following link into your browser: http://bit.ly/SQSIQ6

known to promote heart disease. But maintaining a healthy blood flow is also crucial to optimal brain functioning because the brain relies on a serious flow of blood.

Beyond the critical "rainbow," the brain responds strongly to another culinary group. I hope this surprises you as much as it first surprised me. Herbs—ginger and turmeric are the two big ones—are both potent antioxidants with marked anti-inflammatory properties. Both herbs have anti-anxiety and antidepressant properties and have been shown to enhance longevity. Cinnamon, oregano, thyme and coriander also have high antioxidant properties (sometimes termed oxygen radical absorbance capacity—ORAC) and are highly neuroprotective. Our brains, for all their planet-changing power, are individually delicate. Dietary antioxidants are our most important line of cellular defence in the brain, just as they are throughout the body. Without that protection, free radicals will take their toll prematurely.

But how should we wash down our rainbow of fruit and vegetables and our lip-smacking load of herbs and spices? There is good evidence that moderate red wine consumption protects neurons and other brain cells against cerebral ischemia, macular degeneration, Alzheimer's disease and Parkinson's disease. Ingredients in red wine—polyphenols, quercetin, catechins and resveratrol—have been shown to be protective against neurotoxicity. Specifically, a study done at McGill University in Montreal provides evidence that moderate wine consumption may protect against certain neurological disorders, especially age-related neurodegenerative disorders such as memory loss and dementia.

The McGill team studied cultured cells of the hippocampus, an area of the brain responsible for memory that has been found to be severely affected by Alzheimer's disease and ischemia (poor blood flow) because it is particularly vulnerable to oxidative stress. The results clearly indicated that quercetin and resveratrol are able to protect and even inhibit the damaging effects produced by oxidative stress on the hippocampal neurons that were exposed to the toxicity of nitric oxide. A few other studies have even shown that moderate amounts of ethanol (the alcohol found in wine, beer and other spirits) may have some health benefits, but the deleterious effects of excessive ethanol consumption are all too evident: brain and liver damage and many other health problems.

I personally enjoy a glass or two of red wine but the fermented fruit of the vine can be a double-edged sword unless it's imbibed in moderation. I often recommend that if you don't already consume alcohol, there's no need to start. And according to an article in the *Journal of Agricultural and Food Chemistry*, Concord grape juice may also protect the aging brain. The study found that seniors with mild age-related memory decline made fewer memory errors of a certain type, and had more activity in memory-related parts of the brain, after drinking grape juice regularly for four months. Concord grapes are deep blue to purple due to their high content of polyphenol pigments, the same pigments found in red wine. The study included twenty-one people aged sixty-eight and older, diagnosed with mild age-related memory decline and not meeting the criteria for dementia. They were randomly assigned to receive either 100 percent Concord grape juice or a placebo drink every day for sixteen weeks. The total amount of juice consumed per day was determined by each person's body weight.

The participants underwent memory and mood testing at the beginning and end of the trial. In addition, brain imaging was performed during testing to see if there were differences in activation levels of regions of the brain involved in memory. The

To watch a clip about brain and mood support, scan the QR barcode above into your smart device or enter the following link into your browser: http://bit.ly/LJrgOn

grape juice drinkers made fewer errors on memory tests at the end of the trial and had a higher degree of activation in parts of the right brain hemisphere where researchers believe memory retrieval occurs.

Consuming a "brain diet" to enhance your powers of cognition, to thwart brain disease and to prevent memory loss is only one reason to eat a rainbow, consume spices and drink either wine or grape juice. There's no harm in having better blood sugar control either, or maintaining a lower blood pressure, developing greater nerve cell protection and generally enjoying a higher degree of immunity from disease.

SUPPLEMENTATION: BREAKING THE BLOOD-BRAIN BARRIER

If you're looking to protect yourself from degenerative brain disease such as Alzheimer's or Parkinson's, or hoping to get smarter, or simply seeking to optimize your mood, you'll want to further increase the blood flow to your brain and there are some natural health products that can achieve this. However, we're not talking about just any blood flow. Blood to the brain needs to be rich in oxygen, antioxidants and nutrients. The challenge lies in the fact that the brain is highly selective as to what it lets in. Its primary line of defence is called the blood-brain barrier (BBB).

More than a hundred years ago, it was discovered that if blue dye was injected into the bloodstream of an animal, the tissues of the whole body with the exception of the brain and spinal cord would turn blue. It turned out that in most parts of the body, the capillaries (the smallest blood vessels) are lined with special cells called *endothelial cells*, cells separated by a small amount of space that allows substances to move readily between the inside and the outside of the vessel. However, in the brain the endothelial cells fit tightly together and most substances cannot pass out of the bloodstream into the brain. This barrier is actually semi-permeable, allowing select nutrients such as glucose to be transported out of the blood and into the brain by special methods, while others are prevented from entering.

This barrier in general maintains a *stable* brain environment and protects the brain from foreign substances—including hormones and neurotransmitters that are useful to the rest of the body—because many of these substances may prove injurious. Large molecules for the most part do not pass through the BBB easily, and with very few exceptions only small molecules soluble in fat—about 2 percent—will clear the barrier. These include alcohol, caffeine and nicotine. Most pharmaceutical drugs will not pass—probably a good thing except where the drug can help affective disorders such as schizophrenia, chronic pain and epilepsy. A few small molecule compounds can be used to treat these disorders, but the bad news is that most of them are largely palliative and often have poor safety profiles. Dopamine is an example of a small molecule that is very useful in the treatment of Parkinson's, but has a natural chemical structure that prevents it from crossing the blood-brain barrier. But dopamine can literally hitch a ride on a certain amino acid transporter and sneak through the barrier to provide relief for Parkinson's sufferers.

When it comes to natural medicine, there are a few brain-boosting supplements worth seriously considering. Vinpocetine is one we looked at earlier. A derivative of vincamine, a vinca alkaloid isolated from the leaves of periwinkle (*Vinca minor*), vinpocetine is best known for its neuroprotective effects. It is traditionally used to maintain and improve brain health, cognition and memory. Many of the substances that can increase blood flow in the body cannot get past the blood-brain barrier.

To watch a clip about eyesight support, scan the QR barcode above into your smart device or enter the following link into your browser: http://bit.ly/NNabCN

Vinpocetine is an exception, and can therefore deliver more precious oxygen, glucose and nutrients to our brains. A study in fifteen subjects found a two-week vinpocetine trial enhanced cerebral blood flow, and recent studies using Doppler ultrasound and near-infrared spectroscopy showed enhanced cerebral blood flow in subjects given a single infusion of vinpocetine. It has been studied for its potential to improve attention and alertness, and it may have a positive effect on a damaged brain and on those people who have suffered a stroke. An analysis of six randomized controlled trials involving 731 subjects showed vinpocetine supplementation supported cognitive function. And, where your eyes are extensions of your brain, it is important to note that some fairly well-designed studies show that vinpocetine can also help with poor night vision, glaucoma or macular degeneration. Vinpocetine helps drive production of ATP, our body's energy currency. Who couldn't use a bit more brain energy?

Ginkgo biloba—another well-known "brain booster"—has been used medicinally for thousands of years and is one of the top-selling herbs in North America. The scientific literature doesn't suggest that it busts through the BBB, but it does show that ginkgo leads to an increase of blood flow by inducing endothelium-dependent vasodilatory capacity—that is, it can increase the surface area of blood vessel walls—in healthy elderly adults. Ginkgo has also been shown to benefit people with early-stage Alzheimer's disease and multi-infarct dementia, and it may be as helpful in that application as certain drugs, including the well-known Aricept.

People with Alzheimer's and dementia, however, suffer from far more than just memory loss. They experience varying degrees of irritability, sleep disturbances, depression and more. Though few medications relieve such symptoms to any significant degree, a recent study published in *Neuropsychiatric Disease and Treatment* found that ginkgo biloba might be one more effective natural option. For 24 weeks, more than 400 people with mild to moderate dementia were randomly assigned a daily placebo or 240 mg of ginkgo extract (EGb761). (EGb761 is a product made by the company that commissioned the study.) Participants experienced small but significant improvements in symptoms such as sleep disturbances, indifference, irritability, depression and altered motor behaviours compared with the placebo group.

Other research has reported benefits of ginkgo biloba in patients with symptoms of a syndrome called "cerebral insufficiency." This condition may include poor concentration, confusion, absentmindedness, decreased physical performance, fatigue, headache, dizziness, depression and anxiety. It is believed that cerebral insufficiency is caused by decreased blood flow to the brain due to clogged blood vessels.

Although not definitive, there is also promising early evidence favouring the use of ginkgo for memory enhancement in *healthy* subjects. So, if you would like to *maintain your brain*, you may want to consider supplementing with vinpocetine and ginkgo daily.

LIFESTYLE: FOREST BATHING, SLEEPING AND YOUR CELLPHONE

The words "forest bathing" invite visions of nudes splashing about in a creek deep in the wilderness. Not to say that some of you may not find that a positive and possibly brain-invigorating experience, but I'm afraid that is not exactly what is meant by the Japanese phrase *shinrin-yoku*. Shinrin-yoku refers to a short, leisurely visit to a forest and is regarded as being similar to natural aromatherapy. It is undertaken to achieve relaxation and recreation while breathing in airborne volatile substances called phytoncides (essential oils from wood), which are antimicrobial, volatile organic compounds derived from trees, such as a-pinene and limonene, also found in citrus. Forest bathing trips were first proposed in 1982 by the Forest Agency of Japan. It has now become a recognized relaxation and stress management activity in that country. To confirm what many were speculating, researchers went so far as to bring an instrument capable of measuring brain activity out into the urban and forest settings and found that twenty minutes of shinrin-yoku (compared with twenty minutes in an urban setting) altered cerebral blood flow in a manner that indicated a state of relaxation.

Meanwhile the latest science in the area of forest bathing suggests it can deliver far more than relaxation and volatile substances. It now appears that walking through a forest or naturescape will immerse you in *negative* ions that are very *positive* for human health. Negative ions are charged molecules that we cannot smell, feel, see or taste. The level of these molecules is dependent on the environment that surrounds us. Flora and fauna emit them but they are chronically offset by indoor environments, electronic devices such as computer screens, photocopy machines and televisions, as well as atmospheric conditions such as pollution and air-conditioning. Negative ions are found in abundance in forests and near bodies of moving water but they can also be created by man-made devices including "ion fan towers" and specialized light bulbs. Researchers have linked the abundance of negative air ions that surround us to improved overall health and longevity. They work to promote our antioxidant defence systems, improve mood and enhance blood flow. Perhaps it's time to soak in a forest bath of negative ion bubbles?

But while you immerse yourself in nature, consider turning off your cellphone. The number of people worldwide who are using cellphones is closing in on five billion. Considering that you live in an urbanized world, you're probably one of them. So am I. What may shock you is that the World Health Organization's International Agency for Research on Cancer (IARC) has classified radio frequencies (RF) from cellphones as a "Possible Human Carcinogen" (Class 2B). This is a big step forward in recognizing the serious risks to human health posed by cellphones. However, some scientists say the IARC classification, which only references risk for glioma (a type of brain tumour), is still not strong enough, and that RF should have been classified as a "Probable Human Carcinogen" based on the existing science. Although these findings are still being contested, a series of studies have indicated that cellphone wave emissions, called electromagnetic radiation (EMR), cause biological tissue destruction. And the tissue closest to EMR when using a cellphone is brain tissue.

The cellphone signal is called an "information carrying radio wave" (ICRW) and doesn't exist in nature; it is completely man-made. Since there's nothing like it in nature, when vibration sensors on a cell membrane feel that radio wave, they may interpret it as a foreign invader. We are bio-electric beings, which means we work using chemistry *and* electricity; our brains in particular work this way. Theoretically, brain cell membranes close down pathways known as active transport channels in an effort to protect themselves. They are the same pathways that allow the trillions of cells in your body to exchange nutrients and anti-oxidants. When the ICRW is constant over a period of time, the cell membrane may configure chronically in this state of sympathetic lockdown. When that happens, nutrients cannot enter the cell, and waste products cannot leave. The cell now becomes energy deficient and intercellular communication is compromised. When brain cells can't talk to each other, your brain cannot function as the most important organ, that is, it can't tell everything else in your body what to do. This is clearly a systemic problem.

The consequence of this systemic problem is a compromised immune system, since the disrupted intercellular communication means the signals your cells send out to your immune cells can't reliably get to them either. The immune system becomes less efficient and our bodies find it harder to fight infection. Because waste products aren't moving out of your cells, free radicals build up, attacking the mitochondria (the little energy-producing organelles inside our cells) and interfere with normal DNA repair among other things. The resulting genetic damage can theoretically clone, proliferate and lead to the development of tumours. As a consequence, ongoing studies are investigating whether a brain bathed in ICRW may experience related problems ranging from sleep disturbances, memory loss, focus problems and learning deficits to endrocrine, nervous, digestive, reproductive and immune system compromise.

In the United States and Canada there are well over a million base station antennas that emit ICRW twenty-four hours a day. We are well into a health-risk epidemic caused by the unbridled expansion of wireless communication worldwide that has gone far beyond the mobile phone. You can't go anywhere these days without entering a plume of WiFi or being surrounded by others with their cell phones to their ear. Where many countries are banning WiFi in schools and plaster warning labels on cellphones advising that they be kept away from young children, here in North America we can't get enough of it and "hot-wire" entire cities, "upgrade" virtually every school to wireless while flaunting the all-new and more powerful 5.8 gHz transmitters. Whatever this may be doing to us, there is one sanctuary where we may be able to provide our brains with some relief: our bedrooms. Don't have WiFi anywhere near your bedroom, under or over it, and especially nowhere near your children's rooms. In fact, the best solution is to go hard-wired. Where that may sound difficult and expensive, it is not. It also doesn't take away from the convenience factor and actually increases your Internet speed. Many solutions exist such as turning your home's A/C outlets into Internet connections so that all you need to do is plug your computer's cat-5 cable right into a wall socket and away you go. The other thing you need to consider is turning off your cellphone's mobile network, WiFi and Bluetooth while it is next to you during sleep.

Finally, let me speak of sleep. You need to make optimal amounts of it a priority to ensure that you stay well, think sharply and remember all that you need to. On average, we get nearly two fewer hours of sleep per night than we did about one hundred years ago. The negative effects of sleep deprivation have been known to scientists for centuries, and yet they still haven't conclusively discerned the exact reasons we need the amounts of it we do.

Here's why you want to know in order to stay well. Even tiny amounts of light (including from your cellphone) can suppress production of melatonin, the hormone our bodies make to bring on sleep. You want a dark room. Don't rely on covering your eyes with a mask since researchers have discovered that light will permeate your skin and cause elevations of cortisol that way. Also keep bedroom temperatures cool. You need to have a cool core temperature in order to lull your body and brain into deep-sleep mode. It's advisable to do your workout in the morning since it takes an average of a few hours before your body cools back down to normal temperature following vigorous exercise.

Creating a bedtime routine is also helpful. Setting your alarm at night to signal a time to commence this routine may be just as helpful as the morning alarm. Try taking a warm shower or bath, sipping herbal non-caffeinated tea or doing light stretches. Keep consistent wake and sleep times. Avoid coffee or caffeinated tea after 12 noon. Reading by a dim desk lamp or a softened display screen before bed helps a lot of folks and is generally a better precursor to sleep than the electronic light and often dubious content that floods from the television. If you do watch television before bed opt to set it at a dimmer light emission and avoid topics that upset or annoy you, such as politics, war coverage or disaster reporting.

Bedtime is a perfect time to practise deep, patterned breathing. Take a deep breath in through your nose for a count of five, hold for a count of seven, then exhale through your mouth with pursed lips for eight. Repeat this for several minutes. Doing this whilst also counting backwards from a high number (like one thousand) by increments of seven can be very relaxing—and distracting. It's an effective variation on the traditional counting of sheep and is clearly related to meditation techniques. Busy counting, your brain can't do much else. Sleep follows naturally.

If you are eating a rainbow, spicing up your food, drinking red wine in moderation, using your cellphone with caution and getting good sleep—you are *staying well mentally!*

6. ANTI-INFLAMMATION

DIET: THE ANTI-INFLAMMATORY DIET

Inflammation isn't only the visible, raised, red, hot, swollen and painful symptoms related to arthritis, low back pain, migraines and inflammatory bowel disease. Inflammation is also the underlying, slow and silent cause of heart disease, the fuel behind chronic fatigue syndrome and the mechanism that promotes autoimmunity diseases, to name only a few of its effects. Inflammation happens deep at the cellular level, turning on bad genes that predispose us to everything from diabetes to cancer. By and large, poor nutrition sets the stage for inflammation, so to stay well and maximize our quality of life requires us to avoid any condition that ends in "-itis." You can do that by using the power of superfoods, antioxidant supplements and an exercise routine—one that doesn't promote inflammation.

Chronic inflammation is at the root of most diseases. Consider these facts: one in five people suffer from arthritis, more than 10 percent suffer from diabetes and one in three people will die from complications attributable to atherosclerosis—hardening of the arteries. The common denominator in all these is *inflammation.* Keep in mind that inflammation is the body's response to injury and infection. We can't afford to suppress it altogether.

One way to prevent chronic inflammation is with an anti-inflammatory eating plan that supports your immune system at every meal. Many A-to-Z antioxidants—from alpha lipoic acid to zeaxanthin—help to fight inflammation as well. We'll discuss my favourites a little later on. But it's a major misconception that you can eat poorly and compensate by popping supplements that will somehow give you all you need and magically protect you from inflammation. We've talked about how a healthy diet includes a rainbow of fruits and vegetables, cooking with Asian mushrooms, using less refined foods and consuming much more fibre, partaking of a little red wine (or Concord grape juice), incorporating herbs and spices, and doing our best to keep most of it organic. All of these foods have one thing in common: anti-inflammatory powers.

We've also seen how consuming foods that are rejected by your immune system can contribute to disease, especially when you eat a lot of them. Just a few sensitivities can keep you from feeling your best by causing mild to moderate amounts of inflammation and you want to know what those are if you're to live your best life. Testing for such sensitivities (and re-testing in follow-up) is the only way to understand and manage them effectively. The foods that may show up in your sensitivity profile may be perfectly healthy foods in principle. They may score high on anybody's list of the best and most colourful fruits and veggies. They may be brain-protecting spices. But when it comes to food sensitivities, the issue isn't whether a food is healthy or not, the issue is whether your immune system considers it acceptable. Think about it this way: many people—mostly children—end up in hospital emergency rooms as a consequence of exposure to peanuts, strawberries, seafood and fish—all very healthy foods. Investigating possible food sensitivities remains the best strategy, but until you decide whether to take this approach or not, here are some tips to help you achieve an anti-inflammatory diet.

Tip #1: Eat gritty whole grains. According to the *American Journal of Clinical Nutrition*, processed sugars and other high-glycemic starches increase inflammation. Take them out of your diet and replace them with the real thing. In other words, rather than an oatmeal cookie, have a small bowl of cooked rolled oats. Eating foods that you are sensitive to may cause inflammation and destabilize your insulin and blood sugar levels. A high level of insulin affects cortisol, which causes your body to hold on to and deposit fat rather than allowing you to burn it for energy. The end result: an inflammatory soup. That's why it's so important to swap out sugar-spiking breakfast cereals, bread and muffins that have gluten (one person in 133 is gluten intolerant) for whole grains like quinoa, kasha, oats and brown rice.

Tip #2: There's good, very good, then there's *berry* good. A study in the *Journal of Nutrition* showed that eating berries daily can significantly reduce inflammation. Blueberries, low on the glycemic index, are packed with antioxidants, and they reduce cortisol.

Tip #3: Eat a rainbow. Red radishes, orange yams, purple cabbage and dark-green veggies are rich in vitamin C and other antioxidants that dampen inflammation. Focus on cruciferous vegetables (broccoli, cauliflower, Brussels sprouts and kale), which are also loaded with indole-3-carbonol that helps to protect you against breast cancer. The sulphurous compounds in these veggies help detoxify the liver.

Tip #4: Eat lean protein sources, such as chicken, turkey and wild game. Cut back on fatty red meat and full-fat dairy foods. Meat from grain-fed animals contains virtually no omega-3s but is famously rich in saturated fat. Foods containing arachidonic acid—eggs, organ meats, beef and dairy products—promote inflammation. If you're buying meat, look for free-range livestock that graze in pastures and chickens that have had flax added to their feed, since their meat contains higher levels of omega-3s. When it comes to the best source of protein in the anti-inflammatory diet (assuming you don't have sensitivity to them), choose cold-water fish like salmon, anchovies, mackerel and sardines as they are all a good source of protein and an excellent source of eicosapentaenoic acid (EPA) and docosahexaenoic acid (DHA), the two potent omega-3 fatty acids that can dramatically reduce inflammation. Soy products like edamame, tofu and tempeh are also excellent protein, and when consumed daily (at about 1 to 2 servings) can be significantly cancer preventive.

Tip #5: Time for an oil change. Most cooking and salad dressing oils, shortening and refined baked goods including all vegetable shortening, all margarines, all corn oils, safflower, peanut, and other vegetable cooking and salad oils will ramp up your inflammatory potential. Aside from the pro-inflammatory quality these products have, they are almost always rancid and contain trans fats that are dangerous for your heart and overall health.

Most of North America also consumes far too many fried foods. Cooking at high temperatures is dangerous since oils that are heated to a high temperature become reconfigured, damaged and oxidized, creating toxins and inflammation that are destructive to your body. It is best to bake, boil or steam food and add oils as dressings after the food is cooked.

Avoid refined trans fats and omega-6 oils (soy, corn and cottonseed) in cooking. Increase your use of omega-3 foods and olive oil, which is a great source of oleic acid, making it a powerful anti-inflammatory. Spanish researchers reported in the *Journal of the American College of Nutrition* that people who consume more oleic acid have better insulin function and lower blood sugar. Toss the store-bought salad dressings and opt for olive oil and vinegar, or oil and lemon instead. Add spices and a tiny amount of maple syrup for oomph. That's exactly what top-notch chefs do.

Tip #6: Poach, bake and steam. Grilling creates polycyclic aromatic hydrocarbons (PAHs). Long-term health effects of exposure to PAHs may include cataracts, kidney and liver damage, and jaundice. Repeated skin contact to the PAH naphthalene can result in redness and inflammation of the skin.

Frying creates "advanced glycation end products" (AGEs), a protein bound to a glucose molecule, resulting in damaged, cross-linked proteins. As the body tries to break these AGEs apart, immune cells secrete large amounts of inflammatory cytokines. Many of the diseases that we think of as part of aging are actually caused by this process. Depending on where the AGEs occur, the result can be arthritis, heart disease, cataracts, memory loss, wrinkled skin or diabetes complications, to name a few.

Tip #7: Use more spices to flavour foods. A favourite of mine is turmeric—according to a report in the August 2007 issue of *Biochemical Pharmacology*, it contains many powerful, naturally anti-inflammatory compounds. Turmeric has long been part of curry spice blends used in southern Asian cuisines. Ginger is a relative of turmeric and has its own amazing anti-inflammatory benefits that research suggests might also help control blood sugar.

Tip #8: Go nuts! Where certain nuts are also high in protein and essential fats, walnuts in particular are full of omega-3 fatty acids and, along with almonds and macadamia nuts, are loaded with mono- and polyunsaturated fats that have been shown to prevent heart disease. A big bonus is that nuts increase fibre in the diet, which helps to lower cholesterol in the blood. Don't eat too many though: your own handful (closed) four to five times per week is enough.

But in fact most people don't eat too many nuts. What most people eat too much of are *pro*-inflammatory fatty meats and high-fat cheeses. Ribs, bacon, sausages, hamburger, hot dogs and soft cheeses saturate the North American diet. These high-fat animal foods contain saturated fats loaded with arachidonic acid, one of most dangerous inflammation-causing fats when consumed in excess. It should be noted here that the brain relies on getting *some* arachidonic and it is one of the most important fats in the brain along with DHA, so avoiding it altogether is also unhealthy—not that that's likely for most people. Vegans can consume vegetable oils rich in linoleic acid to increase arachidonic acid intake since

To watch a clip about inflammation support, scan the QR barcode above into your smart device or enter the following link into your browser: http://bit.ly/MAY1wl

a small amount of linoleic acid is converted to arachidonic acid in the body.

Dr Andrew Weil is a medical doctor and integrative health expert. I've followed his work, read his books and articles, and looked up to him for many years. The fact that there is integrative medicine is down to Dr. Weil's influence. He is founder and program director of the Arizona Center for Integrative Medicine, the grandfather of evidence-based complementary medicine and the author of nine books. Dr. Weil has compiled an anti-inflammatory food pyramid that serves as a detailed and practical eating guide that consumers of all ages can use. It can be found online here: http://www.drweil.com/drw/u/ART02995/Dr-Weil-Anti-Inflammatory-Food-Pyramid.html

May I suggest you print out a copy and post it on your fridge? It contains suggested serving sizes and has an interactive educational graphic to help today's families follow the dietary advice that addresses inflammation.

There is another diet that I think is worthy of consideration and it too has credibility as one of the most immune-modulating and health-promoting food regimens discovered. It is called the paleolithic diet, or more commonly the "paleo diet." The paleo diet is also popularly referred to as the "caveman diet," the "Stone Age diet" and the "hunter-gatherer diet," since it is a modern nutritional plan based on the foods consumed by various hominid species during the paleolithic era. It consists basically of wild plants and animals. Hold on a minute, you say. Meat is pro-inflammatory, right? Yes, in the amounts many Western people consume it. But keep in mind that earlier man didn't get to eat it often at all—maybe every few weeks. Otherwise it was plants, nuts and berries for breakfast, lunch and dinner.

The paleolithic period lasted about 2.5 million years and ended around 10,000 years ago. The idea is that the human body evolved over that period of time to adapt to those foods, as our immune and digestive systems learned to recognize and break them down. With the development of agriculture came an entirely foreign group and format of foods. The present-day paleolithic diet consists mainly of fish, grass-fed pasture-raised meats (but probably too much of this compared to what paleolithic man actually ate), vegetables, fruit, roots and nuts, and *excludes* grains, legumes, dairy products, salt, refined sugar and processed oils.

The theory of the paleo diet is based largely in "evolutionary medicine" (also known as "Darwinian medicine"), which is the application of modern evolutionary theory to understanding health and disease. Evolutionary medicine focuses on the adaptation of early humans to their ancestral environment and how those adaptations affect contemporary humans, who eat different foods, perform less physical exercise, practise a different level of hygiene and enjoy a different life expectancy. The logic is that human genetics have scarcely changed since the dawn of agriculture, and therefore that an ideal diet for human health and well-being is one that resembles this ancestral diet. I am firm in my belief in evolutionary medicine, and recognize that the vegan diet does not reflect evolutionary principles. I do, however, believe that the vegan diet can be a useful and therapeutic diet when implemented in the short term (months to years) to fight cancer and reverse heart disease.

Without getting into the complexity in different levels of vegetarianism, it is important to note that *dietary* vegans (or strict vegetarians) eliminate animal products from their diet, whereas *ethical* vegans reject the commodity status of animals and the use of animal products for any purpose. If you look at centenarians—people who live to their hundredth birthday and beyond—you'll note that they have often had little to no access to meat. If you follow Dr. T. Colin Campbell, author of *The*

China Study, he and others suggest that any food with more than 0 mg of cholesterol in it—and especially meat—should be avoided altogether. Another argument for going vegetarian, and one of the strongest, may be that any other way—such as following a paleo diet—is environmentally damaging and eventually (if not already) unsustainable.

Once again, the optimal diet may not be solely what is *good* for you in principle or what keeps Mother Earth in mind, but rather what your immune system gives its stamp of approval to. Food sensitivities can make a health condition worse or simply cause you to experience fatigue, a general bloating, unexplained weight gain or perhaps a depressed mood after eating.

If you determine what you need to take *away* from your diet versus focusing on the fads surrounding what you put *into* it, then you are *staying healthy!*

This planet is home to 7 billion people, for whom there are 7 billion ideal diets. No two people are the same, identical twins included. So, there isn't a single diet that makes sense for everyone. Learning and implementing a diet that doesn't promote inflammation and is customized to consider any potential individualized food sensitivities you may have becomes the *(insert your name here)* diet—the best diet for *you* and the only diet you should be following

SUPPLEMENTATION: THE ANTI-INFLAMMATORY POWERHOUSES

Inflammation is the buzzword of the last decade in medicine, and rightly so. To avoid inflammation is to avoid disease long before it takes hold—nearly every disease science and medicine has discovered. In addition to the sort of anti-inflammation diets I've recommended, certain supplements are known to have powerful anti-inflammatory effects.

Yes, when it comes to your diet, it's a great idea to sprinkle more herbs on your salads, include them in stews and dust them over meats and sauces. But in order to achieve a superpowerful preventive effect, try *supplementing* with them daily—many hundreds of milligrams in each case. It is often a specific ingredient extract that has the anti-inflammatory effect and the nutraceutical industry has figured out what those are, extracted them from the spice and encapsulated them for you.

Garlic

Garlic is well known for its beneficial effect in the prevention of cardiovascular disease and high cholesterol. Regular consumption of garlic (particularly unprocessed garlic) may reduce the risk of developing many diseases associated with inflammation. Garlic supplements that contain standardized amounts of alliin and allicin may be even more powerful and easier to consume daily. Alliin is a sulphur compound that produces allicin via an enzyme called allinase when the garlic bulb is crushed or ground. This compound is also the source of garlic's pungent odour and burning sensation. Other sulphur compounds, peptides, steroids, terpenoids, flavonoids, saponins, selenium, potassium and polyphenols have increasingly been identified as possible active ingredients, the products of metabolized allicin, and all of them work hard to keep inflammation at bay. Allicin is an oily, unstable substance that quickly decomposes, especially at high concentrations. It's important to look for a dried, stabilized extract formulation.

Cinnamon

Cinnamon has been used as a spice in several cultures for centuries. The bark of two species (*Cinnamomum zeylanicum* and *Cinnamomum cassia*)—cinnamon bark—is used as a spice. Its constituents (double-linked type-A polymers and polyphenols) have been shown to have anti-inflammatory, antibacterial, antifungal and antioxidant properties. Studies show that cinnamon is also useful in the treatment and prevention of type 2 diabetes, a disease linked entirely to the damage caused by inflammation. When taking cinnamon as a supplement, use a product that is standardized to a high percentage (10–20 percent) of polyphenols.

Red Hot Peppers

You'd think that cayenne or red hot chili peppers would *cause* inflammation. Their irritating chemicals can certainly burn your mucous membranes if used incorrectly or at too high a dose and, in fact, chili peppers are the basis for the pepper spray that police sometimes turn on demonstrators. The level of heat (pungency) of the Capsicum species depends mainly on the concentration of capsaicinoids, primarily capsaicin. Chili peppers and red peppers come from plants with capsaicinoid levels of 30 to 600 parts per million and 600 to 13,000 parts per million, respectively. Paprika is derived from plants with lower levels of capsaicinoids and is used to flavour less spicy foods, such as ketchup, cheese and salads. Spanish paprika (pimento) is mainly used for colouring. The more spicy chilies, and chili pepper from *Capsicum annuum L.* and *Capsicum frutescens L,* are used in curry powder, hot pepper sauce and chili powder. Cayenne pepper is made by grinding the pungent fruit of *Capsicum* into a powder. A recent Danish study confirmed its ability to suppress the appetite by creating feelings of satiety that can aid in weight loss. And a study done in the UK has confirmed the effectiveness of capsaicin in relieving arthritis pain. Supplementing with capsaicin has been linked to weight loss, pain relief and improved cardiovascular health.

Ginger Root

Gingerol, sometimes referred to as 6-gingerol, is the active anti-inflammatory constituent of fresh ginger. Gingerol is a relative of capsaicin and piperine, the compounds that give hot red peppers and black pepper their respective spiciness. Dried ginger is more pungent than fresh ginger and cooking ginger transforms gingerol into zingerone, which is also less pungent than the dried form. When ginger is dried and encapsulated, gingerol undergoes a dehydration reaction forming "shogaols," which are about twice as pungent as gingerol. Hence, supplementing with ginger is an effective way to stave off inflammation.

Turmeric

Turmeric is derived from the root of the turmeric plant (*Curcuma longa L.*), a member of the ginger family. Curcumin is a yellow-coloured constituent derived from turmeric that the Central Drug Research Institute in India and others have found to be the major constituent responsible for the anti-inflammatory activity. As a strong anti-inflammatory antioxidant, curcumin is most commonly used for joint inflammation and arthritic pain. It can also *prevent* the onset of inflammation, increase energy levels and lower the risk for cancer. A recent University of California study also shows that it may help the immune system clear the brain of amyloid beta, which forms the plaques characteristic of Alzheimer's disease.

The dried root of turmeric is reported to contain 3 to 5 percent curcumin. A review of commercial-grade curcumin found it to contain 10 to 20 percent curcuminoids, desmethoxycurcumin and bisdesmethoxycurcumin. Turmeric may be standardized to contain up to 95 percent curcuminoids in supplement form. Since the majority of research has focused primarily on the constituent curcumin, and not extracts or other constituents of the whole spice, look for a supplement that contains the highest-percent curcuminoids that you can find.

And finally—in total validation of the concept of curry—the healing and health maintenance properties of spices are especially potent when they're combined with one another.

LIFESTYLE: WORKING OUT INFLAMMATION

Nobody doubts that exercise is important. But with the scramble to fit it into a hectic lifestyle, all too often we become weekend warriors: amateur rock climbers, long-distance charity runners, weightlifters—all after our week-long sedentary routine. This behaviour causes alarming amounts of joint and systemic inflammation to occur and can do much more harm than good. So, the question becomes: *how* should we exercise? And, most important, how should we exercise to avoid inflammation?

In order to achieve fitness you need to develop and regularly work on all of your body's physical capabilities, by training in a way that includes aerobic conditioning, muscular conditioning and flexibility. Aerobic conditioning or "cardio" is any activity that utilizes a large amount of oxygen, delivered to the muscles by the lungs, heart and circulatory system. Aerobic conditioning may be achieved through activities such as running, sprinting, cycling, skiing and jumping rope. But the best way to get cardio workouts without mounting up a significant degree of inflammation is to focus on those activities that are non-impactful. Think rebounding, swimming or the elliptical machine—exercises that don't "slam" your joints.

Muscular conditioning is resistance or weight-training exercise and is the single best method to develop and strengthen the muscles. With muscular conditioning, you work the muscles through a *full* range of motion with a focus on both the eccentric (lowering) and concentric (raising) portions of a given movement. The key is not to use weights that are too heavy for you. Use about 60 to 70 percent of what you feel is extremely heavy for you to lift three times. If 100 pounds is extremely heavy for you to lift three times (your "maximum"weight), you might exercise using weights by performing 10 to 12 repetitions of 60 pounds. This approach prevents damage to your joints, extreme muscle and joint tear, and general inflammation.

Most people ignore their flexibility. Stretching the muscles, tendons and ligaments surrounding the joints of your body will promote increased range of motion, decrease the chance of injury and inflammation and improve recovery between workouts.

Excess fat causes inflammation to build up in the body. Most people exercise in order to burn body fat and increase energy levels. This is an important goal in a society beset by an obesity epidemic. Resistance training and stretching are not enough to accomplish this. Shedding unwanted body fat while simultaneously improving heart and lung capacity can be achieved through cardiovascular exercise, but to accomplish this without injuring your body requires a non-impactful approach. And contrary to popular belief, dieting and cutting calories is not the best way to burn body fat. Yes, it's important to eat an anti-inflammatory diet and far fewer refined foods, but it's imperative for your health, energy and fitness to consume sufficient amounts of nutritious foods while exercising your way to a healthier, leaner physique.

Cardio

Most exercise is a form of stress on the body, and inflammation will increase to some degree with exercise intensity and duration—another reason for supplementing with spices. Most experts agree that to further reduce stress and inflammation on your body, it is important to split up your exercise program (cardio and strength) into phases of low, medium and high intensity to allow for maximum recovery and results. Genomic testing can help determine whether your body responds best to high-intensity or medium-intensity exercises. Imagine that—custom exercise plans based on your DNA!

If your goal is to develop a healthy lifestyle, improve your overall health, increase heart and lung capacity and lose some body fat, you need to accomplish thirty minutes of medium-intensity, low-impact activity three times per week. If your goal is to lose significant body fat, forty-five minutes of high-intensity, low-impact exercise is necessary four to five days per week.

Performing your cardio using the correct target heart rate for your body is important to your success. Your target heart rate is the heart rate you'll aim to achieve throughout your exercise in order to maintain your health. You can calculate your target heart rate as follows: from 220 subtract your age then subtract your resting heart rate (RHR). Multiply the result by the exercise intensity expressed as a percent and add your resting heart rate. Your intensity level depends on your level of exercise experience. A beginner operates at an average of 50 to 65 percent intensity, an intermediate at 65 to 80 percent intensity and an advanced at 80 to 90 percent intensity.

Here's an example. Let's say you're fifty years of age and new to regular workouts. When you're still in bed in the morning, count your pulse for exactly sixty seconds at your wrist or at your jaw just below your ear, or wherever you can feel the beat of your heart. Let's say you find your pulse to be, on average and over three days, 70 beats a minute. That's your resting heart rate. These three figures—your age, your exercise status and your RHR—are all you need. Now subtract your age (50) from 220. You get 170, which is your maximum heart rate. Now from your maximum heart rate subtract your RHR (70) to get your heart rate reserve, which is 100. Now multiply your heart rate reserve (100) by your intensity percentage (about 60 per cent, since you're a beginner) to get 60, and add that to your resting heart rate (70) to get 130. So, 130 beats per minute is your target heart rate.

Weights

Walk into any modern workout facility and what you'll see is row upon row of shiny machines, some looking like they're from another planet. Many of these machines can be very useful, especially if you know exactly how to use them. The most useful aspect is usually how they monitor your target heart rate and keep your cardiovascular workout non-impactful. But as far as the weightlifting machines go, most are not necessary. All you need for an effective weight-bearing workout is a set of dumbbells—5 to 30 pounds' worth—and a stability ball.

Humans are designed to lunge, squat, push and pull, rotate their limbs and rotate at the waist. In order to have a well-balanced body, each of these movement patterns should be addressed within your workout program. There are thousands of exercises and even more possible routines well beyond the scope of this book. Just keep in mind that an anti-inflammatory exercise plan that involves a weight-bearing routine relies on the following rules: don't lift more than you can handle comfortably, always learn the appropriate tempo for an exercise, engage in proper and full range of motion, and breathe out on exertion. Should you be able to afford it, investing in a certified personal trainer to guide you along is one of the best things you can do.

You may have heard that you should speak with your doctor before beginning any vigorous exercise program. It is a good and logical warning that I endorse. If you are between the ages of fifteen and sixty-nine, a simple test called the Physical Activity Readiness Questionnaire (PAR-Q) will tell you if you should check with your doctor before you start exercising. If you are over sixty-nine years of age and you are not very active, check with your doctor.

Read these questions carefully and answer each one honestly with yes or no.

- Has your doctor ever said that you have a heart condition and that you should only do physical activity recommended by a doctor?
- Do you feel pain in your chest when you do physical activity?
- In the past month, have you had chest pain when you were not doing physical activity?
- Do you lose your balance because of dizziness or do you ever lose consciousness?
- Do you have a bone or joint problem (for example, back, knee or hip) that could be made worse by a change in your physical activity?
- Is your doctor currently prescribing drugs (e.g., water pills) for your blood pressure or heart condition?
- Do you know of any other reason why you should not do physical activity?

If you answered yes to one or more questions, talk to your doctor before you become much more physically active or before you complete the fitness testing. Tell your doctor about this questionnaire and which questions you answered yes to.

If you answered no to all questions, you can be reasonably sure that you can take part in the following fitness testing and start becoming more physically active. I recommend, however, that you have your blood pressure tested. If you have a reading over 144/94, talk with your doctor before you start any fitness program.

Flexibility

Flexibility is perhaps the most neglected component of the average person's workout, and one of the most important for keeping inflammation at bay. The stretching of your muscles, tendons, ligaments and joint structures is vital for promoting and improving range of motion and will also result in an improvement in the overall aesthetics of your body, increased blood flow to all areas of your body and improved lymphatic drainage, which helps the body to rid itself of inflammation. Additional benefits of engaging in daily stretching include increased physical performance, decreased chance of injury, improved posture and reduced muscle soreness, increased blood flow and an improved sense of well-being. Be sure to stretch lightly before each workout (cardio and strength training). A more aggressive stretch should be completed in the post-workout period immediately following each training session.

Yoga is an excellent practice that incorporates stretching as part of its mainstay. As an ancient Indian system of integrating emotional, mental and physical well-being it is also intended to guide the practitioner along a spiritual path aimed at achieving union with a supreme consciousness. Yoga keeps the body fit and flexible by simply incorporating a series of poses focused on stretching and strengthening while the mind remains focused and quiet. There are a few different types of yoga. *Ashtanga vinyasa* yoga is characterized by a focus on a dynamic connecting posture that creates a flow between the more static traditional yoga postures. *Vinyasa* translates as "linking" and this system also implies the linking of the movement to the breath. Essentially the breath dictates the movement and the length of time held in the postures. Unlike some hatha yoga styles, attention is also placed on the journey between the postures not just the postures themselves. I personally enjoy combining yoga with pilates to get a full workout on days that I'm focusing on flexibility so as to further engage and challenge various muscle groups. Remember that in order to see the benefits of yoga, it is not meant to be performed like a set of repetitions as in weight-bearing exercise. It is intended to be *practised*. Don't worry about how well you do your yoga practice, but rather focus on what the yoga practice does for you.

Besides providing improved circulation, lymphatic drainage and a general sense of well-being, practising yoga has been shown to significantly improve concentration and attention. It is also amazing for relaxation, stress reduction, lowering blood pressure, improving coordination, posture, range of motion, sleep habits and even digestion and bowel regularity.

In fact, besides being a personal practice, some experts see yoga as a complementary therapy to be used as an adjunct to standard therapies in treating a wide range of conditions, including cancer, diabetes, arthritis, asthma, heart disease, migraine and AIDS.

To attain optimal physical and mental function, you should practise yoga two to three times per week for life. Time is of the essence for most of us and finding an hour three times a week to stretch and breathe can be a challenge. But when energy is waning mid-afternoon, consider gathering a group of people in your workplace to do a routine "three o'clock stretch" for fifteen minutes. My bet is that you, your group and your boss will eventually notice increased workplace productivity during that period leading up to the five-o'clock punch-out.

It's incredible how a little deep breathing and muscle movement can completely re-invent your mood and productivity. Let me offer a few ideas for "office-friendly stretches" that will allow you to step away from your desk and recharge. They don't require you to change into your Lululemon or break out the yoga mat, nor do they require any prior experience. All that's needed is a willingness to take a break from hunching over your desk.

Blowing inflammation away

Taking deep breaths ensures that your blood is rich in oxygen. Proper oxygenation to your brain, muscles and organs will ensure that the cells in your body that are in charge of dealing with inflammation can do their job. This particular breathing technique is meant to reduce anxiety and clear your head. When you're stressed out, stress hormones ramp up and their long-term effect is further inflammation, especially to your heart and cardiovascular system. There is no aspect of relaxation more important than breathing, with the emphasis on timing and deepness. Remembering to breathe deeply is like remembering to eat: it can be very advantageous to the brain, like hitting the restart button to restore calm, clear thinking.

To watch a clip about lung support, scan the QR barcode above into your smart device or enter the following link into your browser: http://bit.ly/MjCKVF

Method: Sit in a comfortable, upright position on the floor or in a chair. Inhale through your nose for a count of five (one one thousand . . . two one thousand . . . etc.). Hold that breath in for a count of seven and exhale through pursed lips for a count of eight. Hold that breath out for a full count of two seconds. That's one cycle. Repeat this ten times.

Stretching inflammation out

The focus in each case is to release tension and built-up inflammation.

Neck and Shoulders. Interlace your fingers and raise your arms above your head, with your palms facing upwards. Make sure to look straight ahead and keep your shoulder blades relaxed while your arms remain in line with your ears. Don't shrug your shoulders—relax! Hold for five full breaths in and out through your nose. Let your arms fall down to your sides, roll your shoulders backwards and forwards a few times, then repeat the stretch two or three times, holding each time for five full breaths.

For those pesky and painful shoulder knots, try this. Stand with your feet hip-distance apart. Hold your arms straight out from your sides, parallel to the floor. Bring your arms toward each other, your left elbow over your right. Then bend your elbows so the backs of your hands are touching. Now, hook your right hand over your left so that your palms are facing each other. It's not easy at first and requires some elbow and wrist grease!

Once you have the arm wrap going, look straight ahead and try to keep your elbows lifted. Press your palms into each other while you try to pull your elbows apart. Keep your shoulders relaxed. You should feel a powerful stretch in your neck and between your shoulder blades. Hold for about ten seconds with five deep breaths.

Unwrap your arms and hold them out to the side again. Swing them back toward each other, this time bringing the opposite elbow on top. Repeat the pose in the opposite position.

Chest. Costochondritis is inflammation at a rib junction to the breastbone or sternum that causes chest pain. Many people accordingly end up in the emergency room because the pain of costocondritis can mimic a heart attack. It is often caused from a concave chest due to hunching over a computer keyboard. To counteract this type of inflammation or prevent it altogether, stand with your feet hip-distance apart, reach your hands behind you, clasping them together in a fist at the base of your back. Looking straight ahead, lift your clasped hands as high as you can behind you, pulling your shoulder blades together. Hold for five full breaths.

Back. Back pain is one of the top reasons people see their family doctor. To treat yourself when back pain strikes, try the following: keeping your feet hip-distance apart, bend over at the hip, your head hanging between your knees. If your hamstrings are tight or you've got a big belly, bend your knees slightly. Grab opposite elbows and let your head hang down for five breaths. Stand up, take a few breaths and bend over, head between knees again. To enhance circulation to your head and loosen your neck, gently shake your head "no" and nod your head "yes" as you hang over your legs. Repeat this about three times.

Loosen IT up

After hours of monotonous chair-sitting, you need to loosen up your iliotibial (IT) band—the muscles and connective tissue that is attached to your hip (at the iliac crest) and connects to the bottom of your bigger leg bone (the tibia). To loosen up your IT band, start by bending your left leg, keeping your left foot flat on the ground. Now put your right ankle on top of your left knee. Keeping your back straight and looking forward, push down gently on your right knee with your right hand while bending your left knee until you feel a significant but comfortable stretch. (Support your balance by holding on to a desk or chair with your left hand.) Keep both feet flexed and breathe deeply. You should feel the stretch in your hip and buttocks on your right side. After you've held for a few breaths, switch sides.

It is vitally important any time you stretch to breathe continually whether its "office yoga" or pre-workout stretching. If something hurts, ease off the stretch a little bit and keep breathing. You'll get there eventually.

7. BEYOND YOUR YEARS

DIET: CALORIC DEMANDS

In Chapter Two, we talked about telomeres, the DNA caps at the end of each chromosome. You can picture telomeres as aglets, those little plastic pieces at the end of your shoelaces. Another way of thinking about them—not quite so pleasant—is as bomb fuses. When an aglet wears away, the shoelace soon frays. When the telomeres wear away, the chromosome frays, inhibiting stem cell function, cellular regeneration and organ maintenance, eventuating in cell death and contributing to the aging process. Telomeres shorten over time and research into telomere biochemistry suggests that maintaining their length and health is hugely important in preventing the signs of aging. We saw that you can have telomere-length testing done to evaluate your rate of aging, but if you'd just like to do what you can to live longer, my best advice is to listen to your telomeres. Their tiny voices are crying out, "Hey you! Eat *less* than you need!"

That's right. Even eating at the level of your caloric demands is an assault on your telomeres. Of course, North Americans, along with much of the world now, eat far *more* than the caloric demands of their bodies. Where the average grown male might need between 2,000 and 3,000 calories a day, he is consuming 5,000, 6,000 calories or more a day and is consequently overweight. He's bombarding his telomeres with food. Yet ample research has demonstrated that eating just 200 or 300 calories a day *less* than what our metabolism seems to burn at rest is ideal to slow down the aging process.

The best way to determine your caloric requirements is to have a bioimpedance analysis or a hydrostatic (underwater) body composition test. These tests can discern the proportion of your metabolic tissue (muscle), fat, water and intra/extracellular cell mass. Those tests are hard to come by and most people have to make do with a tape measure, a scale and a calculator. But these tools are enough to assess your personal minimum caloric demands at rest, your so-called resting metabolic rate (RMR).

First, measure your height in centimetres with the tape measure. Next, weigh yourself in kilograms or convert your weight from pounds to kilograms by dividing the pounds by 2.2.

To calculate your daily calorie requirement as a male:

$$(\text{weight} \times 9.99) + (\text{height} \times 6.25) - (\text{age} \times 4.92) + 5$$

Example: if your height is 172 cm, your weight is 74 kg and your age is 39 years. Your minimum calorie requirements are (74 x 9.99) + (172 x 6.25) - (39 x 4.92) + 5 = 1,642 calories per day.

For females, the formula is just slightly different:

$$(\text{weight} \times 9.99) + (\text{height} \times 6.25) - (\text{age} \times 4.92) - 161$$

Example: if your height is 152 cm, your weight is 61 kg and your age is 45 years. Your minimum calorie requirements are (61 x 9.99) + (152 x 6.25) - (45 x 4.92) - 161 = 1,177 calories per day.

As a rough rule of thumb, many experts agree that eating 15 percent less than your caloric demands would be optimal, and starting at age twenty-five (or even a few years earlier) might help to add about four to five years to your life. I must warn you though that this estimate is based mostly on studies of animals and only very preliminary research in humans. And needless to say, eating any amount less than your body needs is uncomfortable. Even if you knew you'd live longer by adopting this strategy, would you spend your life feeling uncomfortable as a trade-off for a few extra years? In the land of plenty, that's going to call for the will of a Buddhist monk.

SUPPLEMENTATION: ANTI-AGING ANTIOXIDANTS

The telomere theory on aging also involves my favourite topic of all: free radicals and antioxidants. Excess free radical activity (oxidative stress) speeds up the aging process and causes telomere shortening to occur faster than it would happen by virtue of normal cell division alone. The former director of the National Institute on

Aging, Dr. Richard Cutler, has said, "The amount of antioxidants in your body is directly proportional to how long you will live."

Free radicals have been studied by chemists since the first one was discovered in the year 1900. In 1954, in the depths of the Cold War, Dr. Denham Harman was studying the effects of radiation on human biological systems at the University of California, Berkeley. He was searching for viable antidotes to the sort of radiation poisoning that would result from an atomic attack. Harman understood that complex and dangerous free radical reactions could result from radiation exposure. He also understood that what made radiation exposure so dangerous was that it triggered the production of the hydroxyl radical, the most powerful and deadly oxygen radical known, one that cannot be neutralized by the evolved antioxidant defence systems of the human body. Large doses of radiation, of course, cause cancer or death, but Harman noticed that mild radiation poisoning produced symptoms similar to premature aging. Since low levels of radical molecules occur naturally in the human body, he wondered if the slow release of naturally occurring free radicals might be responsible for aging and for disease processes. In other words, though radiation-produced radicals were quicker, and therefore deadlier, there might be a connection between them and the free radicals produced by the day-to-day metabolism of the body.

Dr. Harman took the next conceptual step. In 1956, he published his free radical theory of aging, which became one of the most widely accepted explanations for the aging process and it remains so to this day. Harman's theory proposed that a by-product of oxygen metabolism in the human body—those free radical molecules—can react chemically with the molecules of cells and their DNA, breaking necessary links and chains and disrupting structures and eventually bringing about the process we call aging—and ultimately death. What he didn't yet know was that the free radicals were causing damage to the telomere, in essence acting as an accelerant to the bomb fuse. By 1957, Harman had demonstrated that antioxidants, by neutralizing free oxygen radicals, could extend the average lifespan of laboratory mice.

When you supplement with antioxidants (in proper amounts and formats) you are slowing down the aging process. In Chapter Two, I suggested that the concentration in your urine of 8OHdG, a by-product of DNA destruction, has been shown to be an accurate measure of the rate of DNA damage, and that elevated 8OHdG is a sign that antioxidant nutrient intake may need to be increased. Excess free radicals prevent any chance of you seeing a triple-digit birthday and the 8OHdG marker is a good predictor of how many lurk within your body.

Where oxidative stress shortens telomere length and causes the aging process to fast-forward, antioxidant supplements can reduce oxidative stress effectively, which will ultimately improve oxidative defences and mitochondrial function, reduce inflammation and slow vascular aging, thereby keeping your heart younger. Targeted supplementation is key, as antioxidants work synergistically and must be balanced to work most effectively and avoid inducing the opposite effect. "Too much of a good thing . . ." applies here. Overall, increasing antioxidant capacity at the cellular level is critical to maintaining telomere length.

The many ways to slow down your aging

Recent evidence suggests that a high-quality, balanced multivitamin can help maintain telomere length. Specifically, studies have linked longer telomeres with levels of vitamin E, vitamin C, vitamin D, omega-3 fatty acids and the antioxidant resveratrol (the potent nutrient found in red wine and Concord grapes). In addition, levels of the amino acid homocysteine have been inversely associated with telomere length, suggesting that reducing homocysteine levels via folate and vitamin B supplementation may

To watch a clip about anti-aging support, scan the QR barcode above into your smart device or enter the following link into your browser: http://bit.ly/QdLqTw

To watch a clip about omega-3 essential fatty acids, scan the QR barcode above into your smart device or enter the following link into your browser: http://bit.ly/MXakPG

decrease the rate of telomere shortening. Similarly, conditions such as heart disease, diabetes and dementia appear to affect telomere length.

Drown the fuse in oil?

A recent study in patients with coronary artery disease showed a positive association between blood levels of fish oil and a slower rate of telomere shortening over five years. The study, done by researchers from the University of California on more than six hundred patients, found that the higher the blood levels of fish-derived omega-3 acids in patients with coronary heart disease, the longer the telomeres. Add "anti-aging" to the panacea-like offering of omega-3 fish oils!

Epoch: Astragalus

In Chapter Three, I mentioned a New York–based company, T.A. Sciences, that manufactures a supplement in pill form that has been lab-tested and shown to slow the shortening of telomeres. Their product, TA-65, comes from extracts of the herb astragalus, commonly used in traditional Chinese medicine for its immune-boosting properties. According to a study published in the *Journal of Immunology*, substances within astragalus root (called cycloastragenols and astragalosides) can slow the aging process by activating telomerase enzyme production that is responsible for telomere regeneration. There are two patented forms of astragalus root extract, known as TAT2 and TA-65.

Sunshine to slow time

The sun may give you a few more wrinkles, but the right dose of a consequent natural vitamin produced in your body from sun exposure will help you live longer. A study published in the *American Journal of Clinical Nutrition* found that higher vitamin D concentrations, which are easily modifiable through nutritional supplementation and don't actually require roasting in the sun, are associated with longer telomeres. Researchers report that the influence on telomeres of vitamin D is likely due to an inhibitory effect on inflammation as measured by C-reactive protein (CRP), a marker of inflammation.

Reversing age with resveratrol

This compound from red wine has been shown to put the brakes on the aging process. A 2003 study published in the journal *Nature* showed that yeast treated with resveratrol lived 60 percent longer. Admittedly we're quite different from yeast, but more recent research from the Harvard Medical School and the National Institute on Aging has found that resveratrol offers survival benefits in mice—and mice and men are surprisingly similar.

External Armour?

Getting older gradually—and quite naturally—impairs the functioning of cells, tissues, organs and organ systems, thereby increasing vulnerability to disease and giving rise to the characteristic manifestations of aging: loss of muscle and bone mass, a decline in reaction time, compromised hearing and vision, greying of the hair, reduced elasticity of the skin—the list goes on and on. With due attention to our health we can prevent much of this from happening too quickly, but the reduced elasticity of the skin, one of the most observable consequences of the natural and inevitable aging process, continues to evade science. Free radicals damage a skin protein called elastin that holds the cells of the skin together and gives it flexibility and strength. Sooner or later the lack of elastin in the skin will cause it to sag and appear wrinkled and discoloured. If it wasn't for this free radical attack on the elastin, we might be indistinguishable at eighty-five from our high school graduation pictures.

Topical creams loaded with false-hope antioxidants are supposed to slow down the aging of the skin, but few actually do. Their real function seems to be the fuelling of the anti-aging industry. There is however a product on the market that I believe is showing some promise. It is called CIC2 and shows good evidence of slowing the signs of skin aging by lightening the look of brown spots while enhancing skin renewal, resulting in a more youthful appearance. It works using plant stem cell technology. The technology is called "Cellulosome" and *Eryngium maritimum* is the active ingredient. CIC2 assists the process of global skin restructuring and is claimed to regenerate the epidermis (the top layer of skin) and help maintain skin cell dedifferentiation, the process by which a less specialized skin cell becomes a more specialized skin cell.

Smoke and mirrors: hCG and HGH

The global anti-aging market was worth $162.2 billion in 2008 and is projected to reach $274.5 billion in 2013. I suspect more than half of that money is thrown away on products that don't work.

The hormone called human chorionic gonadotropin (hCG) is produced during pregnancy by the developing placenta after conception. In addition, certain cancerous tumours also produce it. The idea of using hCG injections to curb appetite was introduced over fifty years ago and has been carefully studied in over a dozen well-done trials. So, is the so-called "hCG diet"—an ultra-low-calorie diet followed in conjunction with hCG injections—the answer to weight loss and the slowing of the aging clock? No. Every single well-done trial showed that the hCG injections were no better than injecting a saltwater placebo. Of course you lose weight when you lower your caloric intake to 700 or fewer calories per day! If you're strict, you might lose thirty or more pounds in one month. But this plan is downright dangerous and will inevitably cause you to age *faster, not slower.* By the way, this hormone is also sold in stores and online as drops. Since injecting over a hundred international units of hCG is not proven to work for weight loss, drops that barely contain any hCG also do not work—and the drops are illegal. The hormone hCG has never been approved to be in any product sold directly to consumers. Don't waste your money on this one.

Another H-term worth debunking when it comes to living longer is known as HGH or human growth hormone. In children, this hormone is important for normal growth. In adults, HGH helps regulate and maintain tissues and organs. In some cases children whose low levels of natural HGH are impacting their growth rate may receive HGH injections, which is the only approved medical reason for administering it.

A few decades ago, an article appeared in the *New England Journal of Medicine* that showed HGH—a hormone that is made by your body in the pituitary gland—improved the muscle tone and body composition of twelve older men. That tiny piece of research led to an unexpected number of "anti-aging" doctors selling HGH-based supplements to slow down aging, and its off-label use has spawned a multi-billion-dollar industry. Today, the anti-aging industry is riddled with oral formulas of HGH, injections and even inhaled versions of human growth hormone. Studies done since 1990 have produced mixed results. The only firm conclusion is that going to the gym can provide more benefits than HGH (if there are any benefits of HGH at all) with far less cost and risk. Add to that some L-glutamine, a healthy diet and ample amounts of sleep and your naturally occurring HGH will further increase.

As with many hormones, HGH levels decrease as a person gets older. Because real HGH is only available in injection form, it must be given by a doctor. It carries with it some possible side effects including predisposing one to diabetes, swelling, high blood pressure, heart failure and inflammation in the joints. All other forms of HGH are entirely dubious, including amino acid mixes and HGH liquid drops.

LIFESTYLE: DO WHAT CENTENARIANS DO

It is an inescapable biological reality that once the engine of life switches on, telomere shortening, free radical activity and other biological processes catalyze a cellular countdown toward our personal destruction.

If you want to live longer—even qualify to receive a personal message from your head of state—you'd do best to do what centenarians do. Not only do they live to be one hundred years old or more, they usually experience a high quality of life right until the end, defying stereotypes of the aging experience.

Centenarians inhabit a number of "longevity headquarters" around the world including Okinawa, Japan (where they eat many hundreds of calories less than their demands) and Rugao County, a rural community four hours north of Shanghai. Among other virtues such as keeping lifelong friends and eating small portions, they share a very similar diet. These long-lifers eat mostly fish, vegetables, mushrooms, seaweed, corn and buckwheat—and very little red meat. They suffer from virtually no heart and liver disease and have negligible rates of cancer and degenerative diseases. If there is nothing much killing them, they inevitably stick around longer.

Elsewhere, the Sardinians of Italy drink red wine in moderation, share workload in the family, eat pecorino cheese and organic meat once or twice per week. Being Sardinians, they probably consume their share of oily and nutritious sardines too. Meat consumption is low but still part of the diet, which suggests perhaps other factors probably play a more important role.

Eating nuts and beans and observing the Sabbath may also count for a lot—take Seventh-Day Adventists, for example. Many of them live in certain areas in California and have a life expectancy four to seven years longer than that of the average American. They likely live past one hundred because their faith preaches a vegetarian diet and exercise.

Whether your one-hundredth birthday has come and gone as a resident of California, Okinawa, Sardinia, the valleys of Ecuador, the rugged mountains of Armenia or the foothills of the Himalayas, you most likely live in a place with similar environmental characteristics: clean air, good water, organic food, low stress, close communities and unspoiled nature. But the most important and invisible factor may be what the Okinawan centenarians seek out and eventually find—something they call *ikigai.* Ikigai translates as "something one lives for." The French call it "raison d'être." According to the Japanese, finding it requires a deep and often lengthy search of self. The search is regarded as being very important, since it is believed that discovery of one's ikigai brings meaning to life and personal satisfaction on a mental, emotional and spiritual level.

Something that many feel aids in longevity on the physical level is the practice of tai chi. Tai chi is practised by many Asian centenarians and over 100 million people worldwide. It owes its popularity to the fact that it is enjoyable and makes you stronger and more agile. Recent studies confirm that when practised about thirty minutes three times a week, it has numerous health benefits including increased energy, decreased stress, increased immunity, lowered blood pressure, better cognitive functioning, increased joint mobility, an improved cholesterol profile, relief from fibromyalgia symptoms and a better night's sleep. I could go on. It also increases leg muscle strength and provides better balance and posture. Okay, now I'll stop.

It was not too long ago that blowing out a hundred candles on your birthday cake was considered a task you'd never have to take on. Yet with more and more advancements in medicine, with our growing knowledge of telomeres, free radicals and the quenching antioxidants, and with changes in our lifestyles that reflect this new knowledge, attaining that one-hundredth birthday may not be as out of reach as once thought.

Live like a centenarian: Don't smoke, put family first, keep active, keep socially engaged, eat lots of fruits, veggies and whole grains, and, most important, find purpose. Do this, and you're *staying well*—possibly living to a hundred and beyond!

CHAPTER 5

—

CONCLUSION: PAST, PRESENT AND FUTURE MEDICINE

Not more than a few hundred years ago, medical science consisted of a limited body of traditional lore that drew on the available herbs and natural remedies. These might be supplemented by risky procedures and a range of compounds from the local apothecary—most of dubious efficacy and safety. For some dangerous but recognized conditions, terrifying surgical procedures without anaesthetics or antisepsis could sometimes rescue a patient from death—and sometimes precipitate it.

Frankly, we can only be grateful for the evolution of medicine in the last century and a half. But despite these remarkable advances—from heart transplants and brain surgeries to miracle drugs for the treatment of trauma and the prevention of infectious disease—the conventional model has remained ineffective in one very important respect. Our acute-care approach lacks the proper methodology and tools for preventing and treating complex *chronic* disease. The standard medical model, as widely practised, rarely takes into account the unique genetic makeup of each individual, exposures to environmental toxins and the aspects of today's lifestyle that have a direct influence on how healthy we are. In other words, the current health-care model fails to confront any semblance of cause and solutions when it comes to chronic disease.

The outlook can appear bleak, with future generations expected to live shorter and less healthy lives if current trends continue unchecked. What is missing is a model of comprehensive care geared to effectively treat and reverse an escalating crisis of obesity, heart disease, autoimmunity, cancer and diabetes, diseases that (among others) claim the lives of nearly two million North Americans every year. One out of two North American adults lives with at least one chronic illness, and chronic disease already causes 70 percent of deaths each year. There are 81 million people affected with heart disease, 11 million people with cancer and more than one in twenty with depression. Diabetes has doubled in the past twenty years to the point where about one in every three children born in North America today will develop diabetes during their lifetime. Over the last few decades, the number of people in the world with diabetes has increased sevenfold, from 35 million to 225 million.

The shocking reality is that only a few years ago we considered the chronic-disease epidemic to be a "Western world" issue—and certainly epidemiological evidence suggests that whenever people immigrate to North America and adopt our dietary and lifestyle habits, they too develop chronic diseases. But in 2010, 92 million diabetics and 148 million pre-diabetics had been identified in China alone, suggesting a worldwide trend. The inhabitants of the world's four corners no longer have to make the trip to the "lands of endless opportunity" to experience the Western cuisine and lifestyle that contributes to chronicities. Because a major driver of chronic disease is the interaction among genes, activities of daily living, the environment and especially diet, people everywhere are becoming chronically ill as the influence of our Western habits makes itself felt.

I make no secret of my conviction that conventional medical practice would benefit greatly from the influence of natural medicine. There is a plethora of evidence that a huge gap exists—especially in respect to chronic illness—between research and the way doctors actually practise. Most physicians are not adequately trained to assess the underlying causes of complex, chronic disease, or to apply strategies such as nutrition, diet and exercise to both treat and prevent these illnesses in their patients. So even if well-conducted scientific studies showed that, say, a daily dose of mustard could reduce the incidence of Alzheimer's disease, conventionally trained doctors wouldn't know about it because they rarely review such findings in medical journals.

The key to reversing all this is to address the underlying causes of chronic disease: the lifelong daily interactions of genetics, environment and the lifestyle choices of individual human beings. The solution is not only to incorporate the latest in genetic science and systems biology, but to adopt an "enlightened" medicine that would enable physicians and other health professionals to apply individualized-care plans while encouraging patients to take a proactive approach to their own health. Our goal must be to reshape the education and practice of clinical medicine to recognize and validate more appropriate and successful models. As natural health practitioners, our best contribution will be to help conventional practitioners achieve greater proficiency in the assessment, treatment and prevention of the scourge of chronic disease.

There's a problem. My impression is that most North Americans really don't know what to do with the abundance of health data that is now freely available: we may be looking at health information overload. As a result, laypersons are often too quick to accept their doctors' judgment of complementary or alternative approaches—which they usually dismiss out of hand. But if conventional medicine were to pay attention to the evidence-based discoveries emerging from the best of complementary and alternative medicine—non-conventional but safe and effective therapies—and incorporate this wisdom into the mainstream, full and effective health-care reform would ensue.

And of course I can't talk about information overload without mentioning the Internet and the current social media boom. We've quickly caught on to the idea—good or bad—that we can use online search engines to play doctor for purposes of self-diagnosis. In our spare time we can log into Google's Flu Trends, play epidemiologist and take a pretty accurate guess at where the next flu epidemic will hit. When we should be sitting with our family doctor discussing a proposed "wellness plan," we're consulting with Dr. Facebook or Nurse Twitter. Most of us know that the Internet is no more or less than a huge database often riddled with inaccurate information, but we're doing this kind of thing more and more, in part because many, many people feel that their family doctors simply don't take the time to learn about the underlying causes of ill health or how to prevent the recurrence of an illness. God forbid we should visit our doctor and, during the seven minutes allocated to the appointment, talk about more than one part of our body, discuss more than a single organ or delve into more than one issue. How can I blame people for going online?

If you're unfortunate enough to experience a trauma, the place you will find yourself is the emergency room. You're likely to receive miraculous triage and be the recipient of medicine at its best. But let's look at a more everyday scenario: you get sick, you go to the doctor, you get a prescription for a drug, perhaps you get a referral to a specialist, maybe you get a recommendation for further investigation or perhaps for surgery. And all too often, when no diagnosis is arrived at, it's implied that this is another case of "all in your head." Often, that's about it.

But think about it. What name do we give to a preventive approach that honours the body's own ability to heal itself while employing a complementary and integrative approach? We call it "alternative." To factor in our genetics and act to minimize our predispositions, to eat well, to exercise, to supplement, to meditate: *that* we term "alternative!?" To go to the doctor only when we are sick, hurting, ailing or broken in order to receive drugs, surgery or triage seems outdated. I believe it's time for the radical reform of our medical terminology. What we now deem the "conventional" approach is what we really should regard as the "alternative"—an approach to be employed only when and if the integrative natural complementary alternative approach isn't working. The conventional serves best as a last resort if, and only if, we need heroic intervention.

FULL CIRCLE

It was raining that September afternoon in 2008, and I'd forgotten an umbrella. My parking lot was almost a block from the studio so I tried to keep as dry as possible by ducking under awnings and generally jogging more than walking. Not that I was actually late—and not that I was actually nervous—but these were still early days for me. And the guest I would be meeting that day was what anyone in the business would consider "a get": David Suzuki. Not only was the esteemed environmentalist known all over the globe, he had long been a household name in Canada. My viewers at that point were almost exclusively in Toronto. I was highly pleased that he'd agreed to appear on my show, *Wylde on Health*.

My producer, Darren Weir, laughed when I came on the set.

"Okay, Bryce. We're talking environment but you didn't have to bring it in with you."

"Don't worry. I'll dry out in time."

"I dunno. I'm going to ask makeup to bring over a hair dryer just in case. Relax and go over the questions, why don't you."

"How long have we got before we go on air?"

"Over an hour. Relax. You're not usually so twitchy."

"I'm *not* twitchy," I said, but I sat down and did a little deep breathing anyway. I opened my briefcase. I'd announced the Suzuki interview the week before and my viewers had been bombarding me with stuff to ask him. My own approach was pretty obvious. *Wylde on Health* was a health show, and the great man was all about the environment. So I'd be talking about how a deteriorating environment could affect our health directly or indirectly. Simple. What wasn't obvious was how that afternoon would crack open the door for me to a much broader perspective on my medical calling.

My assistant producer at the time, Leila Siu, had compiled a lot of questions from viewers and I wanted these to influence the general shape of the interview. One of the main points I wanted to convey to Suzuki was how strongly I as a health practitioner supported his position on environmental issues. We'd crafted our introduction to reassure him by launching with a criticism of Canadian government environmental policy.

"Bryce! He's here, Bryce."

"What?"

"Dr. Suzuki is here."

The CP24 studio was a high-ceilinged open expanse with small sets and equipment scattered densely everywhere in the semi-dark, broadcasting and taping going on first here, then there. On the far side, I saw David Suzuki striding in. He was a little smaller than I'd expected him to be from TV but the thick waves of white hair were unmistakable. He followed a crew-person across the room and I thrust out my hand.

"Dr. Suzuki. Bryce Wylde. It's an honour, sir."

"Hi." His eyes were sharp behind his wire-rimmed glasses, which were spotted with rain. "I'm ready."

"We're ready too, sir. Would you like to get a cup of coffee and relax a bit? I'm just looking through my notes."

"I'm ready now."

"Well, that's great." I shot a look at Darren, who was standing behind him. Darren made a worried face. "We'll go on air in two hours, sir."

"What do you mean?" Dr. Suzuki looked at me, puzzled. "It's three. I'm here."

"Well, airtime is five, Dr. Suzuki."

"I was told three."

"I'm sorry."

"Have you been outside? I've come over here from the CBC."

"Right."

There was a silence. Dr. Suzuki turned suddenly on his heel.

"I'll be back," he said.

By four-forty, we were a small knot of worried people.

"He said he'd be back, right?" Darren asked for the third time.

"Yeah, he did." Leila was toying nervously with her headset. "He just didn't say when."

Darren ran his fingers through his hair.

"Bryce, look. I haven't even got time to set up an old show as a fill-in. That would take maybe half an hour. If he doesn't appear, you're just going to have to wing it."

"Okay, I'll wing it. What's my line?"

"What do you feel comfortable with? I mean, what can you talk about for an hour?"

"I'll just invite my viewers to get on the phone to me, that's all. We'll talk natural medicine and health. I love that. I'll take any and all questions"

"Eight minutes," Leila said.

On the set just beside us, Ann Rohmer was ready to go for the five o'clock news, live. I quietly took my place in our set.

"I'm pumped," I whispered to my producers through my lapel mike.

"Five minutes," control said. I felt a little shock of something—anticipation perhaps. Was I really ready?

Out of the gloom beyond the lights, David Suzuki appeared.

"Where do you want me?" he said.

"Oh no!" my producers whispered simultaneously through my earpiece.

"Get him miked!" I could hear Darren in the control room hiss at the floor crew over the communal intercom.

"Bryce." Leila's voice in my ear was low, urgent. "I'll load up the original show on the prompter. Stay with me."

We were on air. I thanked Dr. Suzuki for joining us and read from the teleprompter.

"Presidents and prime ministers from around the globe met in New York this week as an opportunity to embrace a clean energy economy and at the same time take responsibility for our collective impact on the environment. However, Canada's prime minister was missing in action."

I read on to the end, then looked at Dr. Suzuki, whose eyes glinted behind his glasses. I didn't see any of the expected warm twinkle thousands of Canadians knew and loved.

"Dr. Suzuki," I said. For a moment I paused. "Dr. Suzuki, do you feel qualified to address questions of climatology when your own background is in an unrelated field. Um, biology, I believe."

Okay, maybe I was a teeny bit flustered. Maybe I was thinking too hard about my viewers and e-mail writers. I probably should have made it crystal clear that my first question was from a viewer. I hoped Raina in Mississauga was happy, because that was her question.

A long pause.

"I believe it was biology," I said, to fill the dead air.

Dr. David Suzuki's eyes, positively flinty, now began to widen. "Who are you to ask me that?" he asked. I instantly wondered the same thing. He shifted to a higher gear. "What background do you have to ask that of me? Who do you think you are, anyway?" His voice was terribly loud. I tried not to look at the camera. "I've got a PhD, my friend, and thirty years' experience. Thirty years!"

To be honest, the man had a point. It was embarrassing at the time but it was as though a key had turned in a lock. It was to cause me to start thinking harder about the perspective I brought to my practice and my media appearances. In the end, it was a terrific interview, though it took me a few minutes to convince Dr. Suzuki that I was on his side, even though I worked for a rival network. But it was this edgy encounter that started me down the path to a realization that the subject of human health was in fact all-encompassing. Up to that point I hadn't entirely understood, except in a very narrow medical sense, the environmental context in which every one of us is totally immersed. Dr. Suzuki, perhaps unintentionally, is an ambassador for how profoundly our health is affected by environmental toxins and destruction. My appreciation for his integrative approach has continued and grown to this day, and I've recently embarked on another book, a tribute to the cooperation of man and planet as embodied in the medical folk wisdom that can still be found in many corners of the world.

Since that afternoon in the studio my understanding has grown, not just of how interconnected and interwoven we are with the exterior world, but of the complex interrelations within our bodies themselves—what scientists are now calling the psycho-neuro-endocrino-immunological web that governs our lives. I've been humbled by the still-mysterious interaction of what we like to call "mind" and what we like to call "body." I've even allowed myself to entertain the idea that somewhere at the far edges of medicine, we may one day discover some underlying truth in Dr. Sha's "energy" medicine. Like many doubting Thomases, I was ready to pass judgment on him quickly that day. I looked for a red button and would have pushed it. I might still.

In preparation for this book, I interviewed Dr. Andrew Weil and I've included the whole interview in an appendix. I asked him, "How does the current health-care system initiate and implement the tremendous need for change required to see North Americans healthy again?"

"The current health-care system is the problem," he said. "So we have to be in charge of initiating and implementing needed change both individually and systemically. First we need a good understanding of what health is. Health is not simply the absence of disease—it is best defined as a positive state of dynamic balance in which a person functions well and interacts with their environment smoothly and efficiently."

His answer sent chills up my spine. Health *isn't* just the absence of disease. It isn't simply about our individual biology, chemistry or genetic destiny, nor is it about what type of medicine works best in what type of disease, ailment or health concern. These are all-important factors to consider. But true health is a balanced interconnectivity of mind-body-spirit-*environment*. Acknowledging this and integrating natural solutions into a system that honours this connectivity is my ideal vision for the future of medicine.

As I grow older, I sense—and I know many have trod this path before me—a unity in things that we who employ the tools of science are only just beginning to fathom. If I could point to one thing that I believe about "future medicine," it is that someday medicine will grasp that awesome unity, and employ it for the benefit of humanity.

APPENDIX

A CONVERSATION WITH DR. ANDREW WEIL

I have been following Dr. Andrew Weil, MD, closely for more than twenty years. He has written extensively on diet and lifestyle, natural medicine, sensible supplementation programs, and effective breathing and meditation techniques. Dr. Weil's view of a better health-care system fully acknowledges the value of an integrative approach, where healing-oriented medicine takes the whole person into account (body, mind and spirit). "Integrative medicine," in Dr. Weil's view, would include all aspects of diet and lifestyle emphasizing the therapeutic relationship between patient and health-care practitioner, while making use of all appropriate therapies, both conventional and alternative.

Not long ago, I approached Dr. Weil to let him know I was working on my second book. Much of it, like my first, *The*

Antioxidant Prescription: How to Use the Power of Antioxidants to Prevent Disease and Stay Healthy for Life, is inspired by what I have learned through Dr. Weil. I recently asked him to weigh in on the topic of health care in North America, and particularly in the United States (where he practises). While some of his answers pertain specifically to U.S. citizens, I believe our lifestyles in Canada are so similar that much of what he says is of great interest to us north of the border.

Bryce Wylde: *When it comes to a collective consciousness around the topic of good health, in North America it seems we are witnessing a paradigm shift. We are becoming increasingly aware that we need a wellness-based approach to health care versus a triage-, resuscitation- and sickness-based model of health care.*

North Americans are seeking preventive concepts, alternatives and complementary approaches to their health. But even aside from the keen interest of the public in the idea of getting healthier, the obesity crisis, diabetes, heart disease and cancer are all testament to our very poor state of health. Since poor diet is so obviously correlated to these problems and in view of the evidence that good nutrition could solve a lot of North Americans' health problems, it is frustrating that on the one hand we're told to eat more fruits and vegetables, yet on the other hand these "commodities" are the most expensive items in the grocery stores. Refined, packaged and processed "foods" are the cheapest!

The question to you, Dr. Weil, is how does the current health-care system initiate and implement the tremendous change that is required to see North Americans healthy again?

Dr. Weil: The current health-care system is the problem, so we have to be in charge of initiating and implementing needed change both individually and systemically.

First we need a good understanding of what health is. Health is not simply the absence of disease—it is best defined as a positive state of dynamic balance in which a person functions well and interacts with their environment smoothly and efficiently. Once embraced, this definition leads to the recognition that each of us is responsible for supporting our own unique and innate capacity for healing. Doctors can help, of course, through the creation of a healing partnership and guidance, but the primary responsibility for maintaining optimal health rests with the individual. You can't afford to get sick, so you have to learn how to make the best dietary and lifestyle choices that can help keep you healthy.

As far as revitalizing our health-care system, there are a number of changes that we can demand immediately, as outlined in my book, *Why Our Health Matters: A Vision of Medicine That Can Transform Our Future*, including:

1) The creation of a new branch at the National Institute of Health to be called the National Institute of Health and Healing, where research into the natural healing power of human beings is promoted and funded. After all, the body has an amazing capacity to defend itself from harm, to regenerate some damaged tissues, and to adapt to injury and loss. We need to honour and better understand these processes in order to develop less invasive and less expensive therapies that effectively utilize the body's healing capacity instead of ignoring it.

2) The creation of an Office of Health Promotion within the U.S. Department of Health and Human Services, where a renewed emphasis on preventing illness and optimizing health can be brought to bear for our citizens. We need to invest real dollars and ingenuity in educating people about nutrition, exercise and other healthy activities. Education is the single most effective way to help defeat the epidemics of obesity, diabetes, high blood pressure and other conditions that lead to life-threatening diseases.

3) The institution of a mandate that insurers cover health promotion and integrative care so that people can learn directly from their health professionals how best to prevent disease, and participate in healthy pursuits such as yoga and the appropriate use of vitamins and supplements. Reimbursing people for these types of activities will help keep them healthy and drive down health-care costs related to the treatment of preventable serious illnesses such as cardiovascular disease and diabetes.

4) The establishment of a Department of Health Education within the U.S. Department of Education so that nutrition, diet and exercise become an integrated part of every child's education early and throughout their schooling in ways that are consistent and innovative.

In addition, the government needs to make it easier for us to make healthy diet and lifestyle choices by subsidizing the healthiest options.

BW: *Apart from the government subsidizing healthy options, it would also make sense to put a harness on mainstream media. These days, TV and other mainstream media outlets influence so much of our decision-making. I think that the government needs to force a censorship on unhealthy commercials as they do on cigarette packages, warnings such as "overconsumption of Twinkies may lead to diabetes." It disturbs me to the core when I see multicoloured, sugar-coated cereals enticing young minds between cartoons while adults delude themselves by watching commercials about happy, healthy people eating a dinner of burgers and fries with their young children in a fast-food restaurant. However, you are absolutely right—the onus is mainly on us as individuals and as parents to distance ourselves from the toxic messaging and ensure censorship for our young children. An even scarier example I can think of is how the pharmaceutical companies in the United States are allowed to promote their drugs this way.*

Pharmaceutical advertising in Canada is heavily regulated comparatively but even here it seems like drug companies are devising ways (such as in "reminder ads" to get consumers to ask their doctors for a specific brand of medication, e.g., "See if X is right for you").

Dr. Weil, in your opinion, how can we lobby the media regulatory boards to stop drug companies from advertising their "ask for this drug by name" campaigns in the media?

AW: The mainstream marketing of pharmaceuticals to the public undermines the doctor-patient relationship, often containing misleading information, and drives the overuse of drug therapy by suggesting that pills can cure all ills. In the industrialized world, only the United States and New Zealand permit direct-to-consumer marketing of prescription drugs. The free market has failed us here.

We need to vigorously lobby our state and local representatives to institute an immediate ban on this type of advertising. As individuals we need to make sure not to become party to the madness—don't ask your doctors for the medications you've seen advertised.

BW: *Great advice. Once again, we all have to wake up and take more of the responsibility. But whether we spend our dollars on nutritious food or fast food, vitamins or drugs, affordability of health care is always a central issue. If the choice is nutritious food and vitamins, then perhaps we don't get sick nearly as often and require far less intervention, but the cost of living goes up. If our choice is fast food and later in life comes the need for drug intervention to reduce a high cholesterol level or if we require heart bypass surgery, for example, then we burden the system tremendously. I think most people get that. But if we are to see a real change happen, we need to effectively exchange a "pay for intervention" to a "pay for prevention" model.*

So, Dr. Weil, how do we convince people to see their doctor before they get sick? How do we convince doctors to sit with their patients long enough to discuss preventive measures? Furthermore, when will available science like gene screening (to perhaps tailor an individualized nutrition, supplement and lifestyle program) enter a mainstream approach?

AW: The current system of health care in the United States is ineffective at promoting the health of its citizens, far too expensive and unsustainable. The health-care "debate" has focused primarily on insurance reform and accessibility, but discussion on the content of optimal health care has yet to begin in earnest. Many experts have weighed in, but I believe that integrative medicine, with its emphasis on diet and lifestyle, disease prevention and health promotion, is the only practical way to transform our health-care system and bring lower-cost, health-enhancing treatments into the mainstream for all to benefit from.

Integrative medicine emphasizes the therapeutic relationship between patient and health-care practitioner, and makes use of all appropriate therapies, both conventional and alternative. Patients will come to see their doctors even when healthy if they understand that maintaining good health is uniquely their own responsibility and that the integrative doctor is their partner on the journey. On the physician's end, my colleagues at the Arizona Center for Integrative Medicine (AzCIM) and I are working to ensure that doctors of the future will recognize their primary role to be supporting the optimal functioning of their patients' innate healing systems, not the management of disease. They will do this by focusing on the individual nature of patients, appropriately using inexpensive and non-invasive means like diet and lifestyle changes first, to both prevent and treat the root causes of disease, resorting to invasive and drug therapies to treat illness and suppress symptoms only when absolutely necessary.

Great progress has been made with genetic testing and its promise is even greater, but genetic testing is a complex issue and far from a straightforward proposition. A significant amount of work still needs to be done before these tests can be credibly used to create individualized healthy lifestyle programs.

BW: *It seems these days that if you ask a medical doctor to treat you without a prescription drug, then they are stumped. How do we educate them to alter their "quick-to-prescribe" approach?*

AW: Western medical doctors have been taught to have more faith in the power of pharmaceutical drugs than in the healing power of nature. An estimated 81 percent of Americans now take at least one prescription medication every day. Safe and effective alternatives to drugs do exist: health professionals should look to them first for managing the most common health problems.

My colleagues at AzCIM and I have developed a model integrative medicine curriculum that exposes residents to new ways of thinking about health and healing. This program is currently in use at a number of medical centres, with the expectation that one day medical schools and residency programs across the country will adopt it. No future doctor should leave training without a working concept of health, an in-depth understanding of the importance of healthy dietary and lifestyle measures, and an honouring of the body's innate healing capacity.

BW: *Absolutely! But this role of invoking preventive medicine that we're discussing here would ultimately lie with the general practitioner (GP). With so many specialists entering practice these days, and not enough generalists, how do we get more doctors to practise as GPs?*

AW: Only 11 percent of U.S. physicians engage in general practice, compared to 50 percent in Canada and 67 percent in Australia, mostly due to skewed pay scales:

internists may make as much as $204,000 USD but a radiologist can earn as much as $911,000 USD. We need to subsidize the training and increase the salaries of primary-care doctors and consider forgiving the student loans of those who opt to become primary-care providers.

BW: *Agreed. Genuine gratitude goes out to you, Dr. Weil, for your time, genius and your ultimate dedication to seeing us all well. Thank you.*

REFERENCES

For a complete listing of the books, article and research studies I relied on for *Wylde on Health*, please visit **wyldeabouthealth.com/books/WyldeOnHealth/further-readings**

ACKNOWLEDGEMENTS

In order to bring you behind-the-scenes on the publication process of this book, I would have to take you through my education at the Ontario College of Homeopathic Medicine, ten years of clinical practice (five of which I also spent directing a large integrative medical practice), four years hosting a television show, years of travel around the world walking through natural health product manufacturing plants to collect the scoop on what works and what is junk, and then walk with you into corporate headquarters of Random House Canada. And there is so much more—but it goes to show just how many people and experiences it took to evolve into this book.

Having written and published my first book through Random House Canada, I knew exactly where my second should be. I'd like to thank the group there who believe in me, and who are superb to work with: Anne Collins, Pamela Murray, Cathy Paine, Marlene Fraser, and especially Brad Martin who, among other virtues, has the good sense to trust Anne.

I want to express my gratitude for the many hours of dedication, incredible insights and creativity to the man who shaped the direction of this book, massaged it through and through, and to someone I can now call my friend, Robert Buckland. I look forward to more adventures together!

Thank you to John Pearce and Chris Casuccio of Westwood Creative Artists for always being there and for effectively "managing my expectations."

I also want to thank the many patients and the thousands of people who sent me questions, notes and emails that inspired this book.

Many of the concepts for the book came to me while hosting the CTV television production *Wylde On Health*, which wouldn't have been possible without the keen eye of Tony Schaschl and Bob McLaughlin, who gave me my first real television break. It became the best-watched talk show on the station because of the hard work and dedication of my production team: Darren Weir, Leila Siu, and Amanda Risser. Thank you guys—together we did some amazing things!

A few important shout-outs. To Dr Mehmet Oz: thank you for always believing in me. I greatly value your friendship and guidance. To Dr Andrew Weil: deepest appreciation for your inspiration in so many areas. To Dr. Tim Cook: you're a shining example of what a doctor should be. I'm proud to know you and practise with you.

If it weren't for the incredible people around me who make up my support team, I simply couldn't get by day-to-day. To them, I submit my deepest appreciation: Frida Ilic (the best PA ever!), Smita Jivan (my ever solid OM), Sharon Feldstein (my mushy manager), Rob McEwan, Caroline De Silva and friends at Argyle Communications (I couldn't manage my efforts without you!), Nan Row (it's gonna happen!), Sunny Raja (thank you for feeding my family such good food!), and my entire panel of experts at www.wyldeabouthealth.com/experts—you're not only there because you're some of the best, but also because you mean the world to me.

Dad, among many other things, you taught that above all family must always come first. If it weren't for the unconditional love of my family and friends, the process of writing this book would have been impossible. To my sisters: My wonderful associate Tanya: we're still on track to heal the world naturally!; Julie, you're my hero—what you've accomplished in the last few years required some strength that I don't know; Merry, I love you equally and always but from afar. Mom—to whom I dedicated this book—thanks for not only making me but also helping to create who I am today. And to my precious extended family—each of member of whom I love very much: the Farbers, the Rosenblatts, and the Rouhis.

To my wife and children: Kelly, Devin, and Zaya. If it weren't for you three, there'd be far less to work this hard for. I live you, love you, dream you, and breathe you. Always have. Always will.

INDEX

BRYCE WYLDE is the author of the national bestseller *The Antioxidant Prescription.* He graduated with a combined honours degree in biology and psychology from York University in Toronto. He went on to pursue a career in complementary alternative medicine and nutrition, graduating with a diploma in homeopathic medicine and health sciences (DHMHS) from the Ontario College of Homeopathic Medicine. Known as a world leader in complementary alternative health, Wylde is a highly knowledgeable and respected natural healthcare practitioner specializing in homeopathy, clinical nutrition and botanical medicine and whose focus is routed within functional medicine. Wylde began his television hosting career with CTV in early 2008 with the highly-rated weekly television show *Wylde on Health*. Wylde lectures frequently on the prevalence of junk science in the natural health world and has made it his mission to "debunk the junk." Bryce Wylde tweets @wyldeonhealth out of Toronto.